RECLAIMING

SOUL

IN HEALTH CARE

Practical Strategies for Revitalizing
Providers of Care

Linda Gambee Henry
James Douglas Henry

Health Forum, Inc.
An American Hospital Association Company
CHICAGO

This publication is designed to provide accurate and authoritative information in regard to the subject matter covered. It is sold with the understanding that neither the author nor the publisher is engaged in rendering legal, accounting, or other professional service. If legal advice or other expert assistance is required, the services of a competent professional should be sought.

The views expressed in this publication are strictly those of the authors and do not necessarily represent official positions of the American Hospital Association.

Printed in the United States of America—4/99

Cover design by Dan Stein

Library of Congress Cataloging-in-Publication Data

Henry, Linda Gambee.
 Reclaiming soul in health care : practical strategies for
revitalizing providers of care / Linda Gambee Henry, James Douglas
Henry.
  p. cm.
 Includes bibliographical references and index.
 ISBN 1-55648-263-9 (pbk.)
 1. Health services administration—Psychological aspects.
2. Health facilities—Sociological aspects. 3. Corporate culture.
4. Medical personnel—Job satisfaction. 5. Soul. I. Henry, James
Douglas. II. Title.
RA971.H465 1999
362.1'068—dc21   98-45909
                                                              CIP

Item number: 001118

Dedication

*W*ith sincerest gratitude we offer our deepest appreciation to the individuals who have served as our mentors. They have challenged us and guided us. But most of all, they believed in us. We warmly dedicate this book to Ruth Tiffany Barnhouse, MD, MDiv; Ernie Bel, MDiv, PhD; Marilyn Crossen; Ira Korman, PhD; Jane McManus; and the Rev. Kathlyn James.

"All things are connected like the blood which unites one family. Whatever befalls the earth befalls the sons of the earth. Man did not weave the web of life; he is merely a strand in it. Whatever he does to the web he does to himself."

—CHIEF SEATTLE (SUQUAMISH TRIBE)

Contents

About the Authors

*L*inda **Gambee Henry** is the owner and president of Marketing and Communication Strategies, located in Kirkland, Washington, near Seattle. She is a marketing consultant specializing in health care and is particularly interested in working with organizations in transition. She has had over 15 years of extensive health care marketing experience within for-profit and not-for-profit organizations in diverse settings. Ms. Henry has served as director of marketing for both small and large hospitals and an academic medical center. As a consultant, she works with hospitals, hospital corporations, medical practices, individual physicians, and dentists. She is an experienced speaker and conducts seminars on a wide range of business, communication, and health care issues. She facilitates organizational strategic planning and assists groups in identifying and clarifying corporate mission and vision. Ms. Henry writes regularly on marketing and business communication, and her articles have appeared in such publications as the *Fort Worth Business Press, PrintWatch,* and *Physician's Marketing & Management.* She received her BS degree from Ball State University. She may be reached at her e-mail address: jlhenry@aol.com.

*J*ames **Douglas Henry** is a principal of Positive Strategies Unlimited in Kirkland, Washington. He has had more than 25 years of experience in organizational enhancement, management training, and career development. For 10 years, he was corporate training manager in Dallas for Texas Utilities, a Fortune 500 company and one of the largest utilities in the nation. Most recently, he served as a part-time career planning consultant for Washington Mutual Bank in Seattle. Mr. Henry's consulting business specializes in strategies for enhancing soul in business. As a consultant, he provides customized training programs and vocational consulting services to groups and individuals. An experienced trainer, he conducts workshops and seminars on such topics as the reenchantment of work, career mission, and building teams with soul. Mr. Henry writes articles on business and vocational issues for such publications as *National Business Employment Weekly, HR Magazine,* the *Kirkland Courier,* and *PrintWatch.* He received his EE degree from Penn State University and MDiv from Lutheran Theological Seminary in Philadelphia. Mr. Henry may be reached at his e-mail address: jlhenry@aol.com.

Preface

$\mathcal{O}$ur book began as the seed of a passionate idea. We didn't realize that its writing would lead us on an incredible journey of discovery, a truly soulful journey. Part of the joy of writing emerges from meeting people we might never have met otherwise. Many of them share our passion for soul, guiding us in new directions. We are immensely grateful to those individuals honoring us by sharing their stories. And we are moved by the depth of their commitment and caring.

This book concerns the soul of health care. It is about purposefulness in reclaiming and enhancing soul in the helping professions. We choose to explore soul rather than spirit, although we view soul and spirit as two words describing the same reality, the whole. They are like two photographs of the same thing from different angles. In many Western traditions, spirit reflects a more transcendental dimension. It brings to bear more of a masculine energy, of a more doing rather than a being, whereas soul inclines more toward the feminine, as in Mother Earth. Soul grounds itself in the vernacular. "Just as there are spiritual practices in search of the highest and most refined reaches of human potential," writes Moore, "so there is soul practice in pursuit of the juices and nutriments of life's entanglements."[1]

We choose to write more about soul because many people, and particularly health care professionals, need to slow down at times. Among other things, soulfulness involves taking time to meaningfully connect to one another. It includes using our senses to enjoy ordinary life, including music, art, and nature. Soul often guides us into reflection, into a stance of not doing. And anyway, what is the meaning behind what we do? How does it affect the sacredness and quality of life?

In his book *Time and the Soul,* Needleman reports the story of having dinner with a brilliant and devoted doctor. As the two of them reflect about the meaning of time, the physician laments:

> You don't understand. I have no time! I am pathologically busy. It's beyond anything I have ever imagined . . . more and more people depend on me. More and more things, good things, important things, keep coming to me. Any one of them is worth the whole of my attention and needs my time. But ten, twenty of them? A hundred of them? And it is the same with my staff. They are all being driven past their limits.[2]

Like this doctor, health care professionals may need to retreat to the roots of the profession, reclaiming its original soul, renewing its energy.

References

[1] Thomas Moore, *Soulmates* (New York: HarperCollins, 1994), p. 16.

[2] Jacob Needleman, *Time and the Soul* (New York: Currency/ Doubleday, 1998), p. 60.

Acknowledgments

If we were to acknowledge everyone who has helped and supported us in this task, it would require another chapter! To those who shared their stories and their passion, we are immensely grateful. For the support and encouragement of our family, friends, and colleagues, our heartfelt thanks.

In particular, we would like to express our appreciation to each of the following who have made this book possible. We are deeply indebted to our editor at AHA Press, Rick Hill, for his enthusiastic support; Emily-Mae Stafford for reviewing original drafts; the Shared Journey group for sharing and enriching our lives; Ethel McAfoose, for her long-time support and friendship and for reading early chapters; Jody Carona, Vicki Brown, Leah Kliger, and Michael Handley for their personal and professional contributions; Margaret McGovern for participating in the original conceptualization of the four qualities of soul in organizations; and the Alliance for Healthcare Strategy and Marketing, whose belief in the original presentation material was the book's catalyst. We say many, many thanks.

Introduction

$\mathcal{A}$s we approach the end of the millennium, many of us struggle to grasp and reorient ourselves toward an earlier perception of the nature of the universe. It is a perception being revitalized by a growing number of scientists, especially quantum physicists. The world is not a machine but rather a tapestry of relationships. As Chief Seattle of the Suquamish tribe suggests, we are all strands woven into the fabric. According to this world view, everything we do affects everything and everyone else, including having our actions turn back upon ourselves.

Perhaps this is why, almost instinctively, physicians are warned from the beginning of medical school to do no harm. Stated in a more positive manner in the Hippocratic oath, "In every house where I come I will enter only for the good of my patients."

WHY RECOVERING SOUL IN HEALTH CARE?

$\mathcal{O}$ur interest in the mysterious subject of soul is, in part, a story of our own journeys in health care and business. Because we as a couple have traveled different roads, this book represents the culmination of our experiences and understanding. Some of you may find similarities in your own history; others may simply relate to this topic through personal knowledge or stories shared by friends and associates.

Over the years, without understanding what it was, it was obvious to us that some organizations are filled with an atmosphere that welcomes its patients and customers. These groups respect their employees and invite them to participate in activities crucial to the organization's success. This atmosphere and the sense of connectedness among the internal staff cannot be defined in words. It appears to be mysterious, yet it is the essence of the organization: it is what we have come to call its *soul*. In contrast, there are also organizations that convey an atmosphere of distrust, of disrespect, with an attitude that people are expendable commodities; these organizations have diminished *soul*.

We trust this book will be a guide for enhancing the helping professions. Although we discuss current, traumatic changes, calling on personal experiences and those of many others, our intent is to report the best of what is. In *The Thin Book of Appreciative Inquiry,* Hammond states, "By paying attention to problems, we emphasize and amplify them. This approach is consistent with the historical attitude in American business (and health care) that sees human systems as machines and parts (people) as interchangeable."[1] In contrast, by addressing the best of what is, we honor and enhance the soul of the profession.

OUR AUDIENCE

*W*e believe that any health care professional who is involved in providing direct care or who has managerial or support responsibilities will benefit from understanding the qualities of the *soulful organization*. Such professionals may be found in acute care settings, mental health facilities, extended care facilities, and similar environments. They include such people as physicians, administrators, department managers, human resources staff, marketing/public relations professionals, continuing education staff, and adjunct health care practitioners.

What This Book Is and Is Not

Reclaiming Soul in Health Care is not a 12-easy-steps approach to the soulful organization. Nor is it a discourse on the philosophical nature of soul. Rather, it applies the ideas of those who are committed to enhancing soul in the business environment and adapts these perceptions of soul to health care. It is intended as a practical guide to help readers gain an awareness of the relationship between soul and a profitable organization. It reframes the weighty and philosophical concepts of soul into everyday business language and activity. It offers dozens of practical, low-cost suggestions for enhancing soul.

This book is also an invitation to individuals to begin soul-searching so as to understand why we want to become involved and what difference it makes to us. We hope this book will encourage readers to converse with others in their organizations, to engage in "what if" scenarios. And, finally, we challenge readers to develop their own action plans for making a difference.

> *"At the systemic level, the soul of health care will only be restored to the degree that each individual takes responsibility to embody soul personally. . . . We cannot afford to go forward building bigger and more dehumanizing systems as if soul did not matter. . . . With compassion at the center of each person's spirit, we have hope of creating life-giving health care systems."*[2]
>
> —Marie Morgan
> and Mark Leavitt
>
>

We believe what distinguishes this book is that it introduces a distinct kind of vocabulary, a fresh way of using language that allows us to speak of experiences in a much more sacred manner. We explore what soul is and the difference that being a soulful organization makes to employees, to customer/patient satisfaction, and ultimately to the bottom line.

CHAPTER HIGHLIGHTS

Chapter 1: The Journey Begins. We begin with our own stories and explain how most of us instinctively know when we participate in a soulful organization, perhaps without ever using the word *soulful.* In a similar manner, we know when soul is being diminished.

Chapter 2: The Nature of Soul. Mysterious and beyond definition, soul is like a living organism, an unbounded cosmic web embracing everyone and everything. It stands in contrast to the common Western perception of the world as a machine. Images of soul emerge from the Saxon word *hal,* from which also come the words *healing* and *wholeness.*

Chapter 3: Soul—The Missing Dimension in Health Care. Today the health care professions continue to experience chaotic and ongoing change. Many physicians face loss of mission, autonomy, and income. Patients receive visits from the "one-minute doctor." Many employees are overworked and yet wonder about job security.

Chapter 4: Paradigm Shift. We are moving from the industrial age to the information age where the machine metaphor for how we see the world no longer works. Here, the emphasis must shift to soul and the web of connectedness, caring, and compassion. The new paradigm encourages a partnership between patient and health care provider and affects our relationship to work.

Chapter 5: Soul and Individuality. A soulful personality is multifaceted. The more we individuate, establishing unique identities, the more we connect to soul. To be human is to have a particular story. A pot of gold awaits us even on the shadow side of our personality.

Chapter 6: Soul and Vocation. Just as an acorn knows instinctively what it means to become an oak tree, so we have a vocational calling.

It is to use our unique gifts through health care and other professions to contribute to the needs of the world. One's personal career mission can be aligned with an organization's mission.

Chapter 7: Soul and Diversity. Biodiversity serves as the key to the maintenance of the world. The health care professions prosper in this diversity. Even our inner, psychological makeup is diverse. In particular, each person's masculine and feminine energies, when appreciated and working in harmony, produce enormous creativity and synergy $(1 + 1 = 3)$.

Chapter 8: Soul and Community. Like high-flying geese, soulful work communities embody a shared vision, respect, trust, and high levels of mutual sharing and caring. One strategy for reclaiming soul in health care involves exploring and amplifying the best of what is in the organization.

Chapter 9: Applications of Soul in Organizations. Here, numerous examples of soul in non–health care and health care organizations are highlighted. They bear testimony to the fact that enhancing soul produces positive, bottom-line results.

Chapter 10: Developing Strategies for Reclaiming Soul. A simple, logical, practical change model is introduced. It is used to identify positive and negative forces affecting health care professionals, their organizations, and their missions. A cafeteria menu of strategies gives our readers dozens of no-cost or low-cost suggestions for enhancing soul in the organization.

References

[1] Sue Annis Hammond, *The Thin Book of Appreciative Inquiry* (Plano, Tex.: Kodiak Consulting, 1996), p. 6.

[2] Marie Morgan and Mark Leavitt, "Recovering the Soul of Health Care," in *Rediscovering the Soul of Business, A Renaissance of Values,* eds. Bill De Foore and John Renesch (San Francisco: Sterling & Stone, 1995), p. 338.

CHAPTER ONE

The Journey Begins

"The twenty-first century will be anything but
business as usual. Institutions . . . must honor
the souls of the individuals who work for them
and the great soul of the natural world."[1]

—David Whyte

EXPERIENCES IN HEALTH CARE (LINDA'S STORIES)

My mother lay dying in the sterile, white hospital bed that looked too large to hold her shrinking body. Racked by pain in the advanced stages of cancer, she had elected to die. She, who had feared death, who had avoided even talking about its inevitability, decided to stop eating, rejecting the feeding tube that would prolong her life.

Having worked within the health care industry all of my adult career, I was not intimidated by the inner workings of the hospital nor by its medical and nursing staff. I was torn, though, by being both a family member—angry, grieving, frustrated, and helpless— and by being the "professional." A part of me seemed to function as though I were "one of them" and to feel apologetic when my mother's needs did not fit within the boundaries of their orderly schedule. When aides stood outside her door laughing and talking loudly about their dates, I felt embarrassed and thought I should apologize for her when she became agitated and asked them not to stand there. After all, she was dying; they were living. The consulting specialist monitoring her pain medication was reluctant to increase her dosage to offer more comfort. He could not admit that she was, in fact, dying and did not want to run the risk of addiction. I didn't fight as much as I might have for its increase.

The clinical professionals were skilled and efficient, but many staff members who could have made a difference and had an opportunity to connect with my mother didn't bother. She was the dying patient, the one with metastasized cancer who was outstaying her "disease-related group's" specified length of stay. Luckily, our family members who were on staff in clinical and managerial positions helped considerably, or there would have been even fewer instances of compassionate connecting.

MORE STORIES

*C*ontrast this picture with the following scenario. The woman lay in the hospital bed dreading the upcoming tumor biopsy. She firmly believed the tumor was malignant and feared hearing a diagnosis of cancer.

The nurses and doctors were competent and caring, and their attitude was reflected in the action of the employee who made the biggest difference—the housekeeper. Every day that she was on duty and came to the room to clean, she would visit with this woman, listening, empathizing, comforting. It was not her job, yet she felt connected to the healing mission of the hospital; to her it *was* part of her job. And though she was not working on the day of the biopsy, she came by to see how the surgery had gone and then rejoiced with the patient when she learned the tumor was benign.

It is not unusual for Madison Regional Medical Center (the name has been altered) to attract patients and visitors from down the street or from out of the country. Walking in the door of this large facility, one immediately is struck by the warmth and concern of the various clinical and support staff. Whether it is the volunteers who staff the information desk and deliver the flowers, the nurses who care for the routine medical cases or the more difficult and complex patients, or the staff who assist the out-of-town families with their travel and housing needs, there is a feeling of warmth, caring, and concern.

St. John's Memorial Hospital (again the name has been changed) is a medium-sized facility with an excellent reputation for its medical care. Walking in its main entrance, one feels that "something" is not quite right here. The atmosphere seems cold. Employees are fairly somber and their overheard conversations reveal discontent with a recent management decision. There is little interaction with visitors or apparent interest in helping people who appear lost or confused. The signage is either lacking or confusing. The patient check-in area is small and staffed by individuals who are not knowledgeable. The general atmosphere and unwelcoming attitude make a confused visitor feel like an intruder in the day's business.

What are the differences between the four examples above? Each is a good hospital medically. All have competent and professional staff. Yet in Madison Regional, there is an atmosphere of warmth and caring, where people respond to a patient's or visitor's needs whether or not it's their job. Similar facilities resonate with a presence; they exude a mysterious something that is palpable and obvious, though it may not be identified in so many words.

And then there are other hospitals and medical practices similar to the first example and to St. John's that convey an atmosphere of distrust and a disrespect of others. People often are treated as though they were expendable commodities. There is a disconnection with employees. Visitors and even patients may be viewed by staff as annoyances in the daily order of things and accepted only when they fit into a convenient schedule.

I have had experience, as a professional and as a family member, with hospitals like those in the first and fourth example. But over the years as a marketing professional, I have also worked with other organizations that, internally and externally, respected their employees. The mysterious ingredient that characterizes the latter kinds of organizations is the essence of such organizations—their soul. And such organizations are considered soulful.

EXPERIENCES IN NON–HEALTH CARE (JIM'S STORIES)

*I*n the early 1970s I was burned out as a caregiver in a not-for-profit, service-oriented institution. After a grueling, anxiety-ridden 10-month career transition and job search, I began a new job as a training specialist in a business enterprise with fresh energy, expecting to revitalize my career and make a significant contribution.

Within a month or so, however, I was discontented and began questioning the wisdom of my move. My boss, while pleasant enough, was extremely conservative, mirroring the culture of the overall organization. No significant projects or tasks loomed on the horizon. Internal communication was largely limited to memos written according to detailed guidelines, including margins and spacing.

Status and reporting levels determined office space, with executives located on the top floor. The dress of the day was largely gray conservative suits. Most managers had secretaries, and all secretaries were white females. In fact, ethnic minorities were found primarily in custodial jobs.

Any display of emotion, positive or otherwise, was limited to professional football or baseball, and celebrations were rare, apart from the annual quarter-century club banquet, at which time the president recited a slightly modified version of the previous year's homily.

Individuality and diversity were almost nonexistent, and creativity was contained within tight boundaries. Most employees assumed that the work was uninspiring and boring, and employees were not assigned jobs according to their skills and aptitude. Engineers and accountants, for example, were often assigned to the personnel department; and sometimes personnel employees were assigned to management positions in other departments with a make-it-or-break-it attitude.

This was my first experience with soul—actually its lack—in the world of business. Soul was not entirely absent, however. Measured against the four primary qualities of a soulful organization discussed later, on a scale from 1 to 10, with 10 being a uniquely soulful organization, this company would probably have scored a 2 or 3.

THE SCENE CHANGES

About 25 years later, from the mid- to the late 1990s, I worked for a major financial institution as a career planning specialist in human resources. This organization "walked the talk" when it came to diversity. My boss was female, as was her manager. I had African- and Mexican-American associates as well as gays and people of various ages. In fact, I was 59 years old when I was hired.

When I began work, my manager laid out her expectations for me as well as what I could expect from her. Work was to be accomplished independently and professionally, with goals established according to my clients' needs and by departmental consensus. I was expected to be creative and innovative. In fact, I was hired in part because of examples of my creativity that I shared during the interview process.

There were no secretaries and few office assistants; everyone performed his or her own administrative work. Office space was determined by need and availability. In fact, at one point my office measured roughly twice that of my manager's and had twice the window space. I individualized my office space to reflect soulful activities and memories, both on and off the job. Whenever appropriate, my clothes reflected my personality and particular tastes, and "dress down" was allowed every Friday.

Within several months of my arrival, members of my team completed a series of career assessment instruments. Composite information about vocational interests, personality strengths, key functional skills, and work values was shared. This information was then used by my manager and peers when we worked on special projects and tasks.

During the ensuing months, a deep sense of community emerged. Many team members became friends both on and off the job. Monthly staff meetings often began with a roundtable report of what was going on in our lives. Birthdays and holidays were celebrated regularly, and everyone was allowed on one occasion to attend the state fair. I believe this organization, on a scale of 1 to 10, would rank at least an 8 in terms of the quality of soul in its business and caregiving. What, then, is soul?

Reference

[1] David Whyte, *The Heart Aroused* (New York: Currency Doubleday, 1994), pp. 10–11.

CHAPTER TWO

The Nature of Soul

*"The soul itself is a mystery and therefore has
great respect for the inexplicable. Don't try to
figure everything out."*[1]

—Frederic and Mary Ann Brussat

*P*erhaps you've experienced firsthand as a patient the sense of caring and empathy so important to healing. Possibly you were a family member needing the reassurance that your hospitalized loved one was in good hands when you were absent from the bedside. Or, as a staff member, you may have felt you were part of something broader than the narrow boundaries of your usual roles. And it's possible for you to feel this way even without having clinical responsibilities.

HOW DO WE DEFINE THIS MYSTERIOUS SOMETHING CALLED SOUL?

*N*ot long ago, a number of health care marketing professionals were asked to tell what soul meant to them using a key word or phrase. The words selected conveyed a sense of emotion: depth, passion, core presence, spirit, love, connections. Regardless of their response, all agreed that soul depicts the core essence of something.

Many of us relate mission to calling. We may talk about some-one's vocational calling—that is to say, their career mission in life. Likewise, we see an organization's mission as being that which it is called to do—its business, or its core essence. Therefore, the soul of an organization may be likened to its mission, its center. And mission must express not only *what* it is about, but *how* it will do it. In health care, the core business historically has been promoting health and healing. Therefore its mission—health and healing—is its core or soul.

A number of physicians were among the health care profession-als interviewed for this book. Perhaps not surprising was the depth of their emotion and their intense feelings associated with the soul and mission of working with patients. A physician who began her career in medicine some years ago and specializes in reproductive medicine defined health care's mission as the "working together [physician and team] to help others." Reflecting on what soul means to her as a physician, she says, "Trying to help them [patients] with a problem can be a very satisfying experience . . . with all members [of the team] involved . . . and when a physician does that to care for the patient, I think [that] has a lot to do with what you are describing as soul in health care. It's one of the most satisfying things that you can do ever."

One internal medicine practitioner passionately discussed this issue: "It is a privilege for me to get to know (talk to) patients in a way that most people do not get to do." Still another view was shared by a senior lecturer in the department of medical history and ethics of a prestigious medical school. He believes soul is reaching for the human connection.

In the anthology *Rediscovering the Soul of Business, A Renaissance of Values,* Morgan and Leavitt state: "Soul is that hard-to-define but easy-to-recognize quality at the heart of what it means to be human. I would contend that health care is unhealthy without the component of soul. . . . The soul in health care—a lot of the 'magic' of the whole process—is in the people and relationships, just as much as it is in the treatments, the drugs, the surgeries, the brilliant technologies."[2]

Soul As Mystery
In his book *Care of the Soul*[3] and in his many other offerings, Moore emphatically claims that soul is beyond definition. *Soul is a mystery.* Derived from the Latin word *misterium,* mystery alludes to a truth incomprehensible to full understanding. It reflects that which remains concealed from full knowledge or view, that which inspires wonder.

People need mystery. It captivates the mind and stimulates the imagination. If there is no wonder, there is nothing holy. Without surprise, life would be unbearably dull. Mystery is one of the reasons why millions of people participate in religious activities and rituals of one kind or another. In a linear, reason-based world of information and gadgetry, the current interest and revitalization of spirituality is certainly powered in part by a need for mystery.

> *"The first mystery is simply that there is a mystery. / A mystery that can never be explained or understood. / Only encountered from time to time. . . ."*[4]
>
> —Lawrence Kushner
>
>

The last time we visited a hospital unrelated to business was to celebrate the birth of a granddaughter. Within the hour of her arrival, we delighted in the marvel of holding Sarah in our arms. We experience soul most deeply during times like this, especially at the extremities of life, during birth and death. No wonder we conduct some of our most significant rituals around these events. They engage us in wonder and mystery.

Undoubtedly, many physical, mental, and social health care professionals gravitate to their fields because of a compelling desire to research mystery. Many of these vocations are by nature investigative, searching to understand the nature of health and the reasons for affliction. Obviously, solving the mystery of disease is an ongoing challenge. Even for those not involved on a daily basis with this task, there is often a feeling of being connected to the healing arena.

Soul As a Living Organism

If soul is mysterious, then we must talk around it, using the language of simile and metaphor. Simile suggests that something *is like* something else. Metaphor reminds us that something acts *as if* it were something else. For example, the Swiss psychologist Carl Jung constructed many of his formulations around the image of soul as a unifying energy. Soul is like energy. Or to describe it in metaphorical terms, soul acts as if it were a living, energized organism, a perception that gives weight to the ancient instruction that "the soul is not in the body, but the body is in the soul."

In the second chapter of Genesis, the Hebrew word generally used for soul is *nephesh,* meaning "living being." "Then the Lord God formed man of dust from the ground, and breathed into his nostrils the breath of life; and man became a living being [*nephesh*]" (Gen. 2:7 RSV). Here we observe the intimate connection between soul and health care, for the latter is intrinsically involved in keeping people healthy and alive.

We also observe the relationship between soul and organization. An organization implies a system of people, things, processes, and connections operating (we hope) as a unified entity for a particular purpose. It functions like the human body, which involves the heart, lungs, liver, stomach, and so on, operating as a unified system. Like the body, an organization is not functioning properly if it is dysfunctional or diseased. We could say that the soul of that group is diminished or forsaken. The institution is wounded; its energy is sapped and its life in jeopardy.

Quite often, unfortunately, especially during mergers, acquisitions, and reorganizations, organizations operate in a dispassionate, cold, impersonal, and cruel manner. Almost all of us have personally experienced or have heard horror stories of how employees receive a pink slip. During such times, we might refer to the soul of the organization as being "iced over."

Many individuals in health care chose the healing profession because they wanted to make a difference in people's lives. They joined organizations whose perceived mission was that of healing—solving the mystery of disease and illness. When organizations aren't functioning properly, many health care professionals become frustrated by the incongruity they see between the mission of healing and the actions of their organizations.

> *"Soul is at the center of the business enterprise. If you nurture the soul of business, not only can you compete with the biggest players in the game, you will add a real meaning to your work and make a real contribution to society."*[5]
>
> —Tom Chappell, president of Tom's of Maine

In reflecting on her early days in practice, one physician related firsthand the loss of soul within a large, established hospital in the Northwest. "When I first came here I had a good sense of relating with other physicians—everyone seemed to be working together. People felt valued—even those pushing the gurneys. There was soul. Not now." She believes a series of financial changes and reorganizations resulting in staff reductions that were not handled in a caring and humane manner did much to diminish the feeling of soul.

"Today, I realize that I can't relate to the big organization; I can't really do anything about its changing. My world has to be my own practice and keeping my employees happy. When they are happy and we work as a team—really being connected to the greater mission—then I can do my work."

Soul and the Whole

Other images commonly used to understand the nature of soul emerge from the word *whole.* The word *health* comes from the Saxon word *hal,* which is also the origin of the word *whole.* When we say "hello" to someone, we are wishing that person health and well-being.

Carl Jung in particular liked to associate wholeness with soul. It represented his way of describing soul as magnificently unbounded. Soul is at the same time the outside-outside of the universe and the inside-inside of all reality. Soul is the whole. The failure to consider the soul or entirety of a person during the treatment of a disease would, according to Jung, contradict the essence of health care.

> *"Soul is not just a place in Korea."*
>
> —Anonymous
>
> ❧

The Greek word for soul is *psyche,* as in psychology. Greek mythology introduces us to the story of Psyche, a maiden who was loved by Eros and who eventually was united with him. Psyche subsequently became the personification of soul. As we shall see later, soul possesses some distinctly feminine qualities. In any case, in the generic sense of the word, psychology is the study of the soul, or of the whole. The proper translation of *psychotherapy* from the Greek is "pay tribute to the soul." Of course, it may be safe to assume in our time that not too many psychologists are students of the soul.

The mandala captured Jung's attention as a universal symbol of soul or wholeness. It comes in countless shapes and forms, although the mandala in figure 2-1 represents a kind of generic image. It is a quadrated circle embracing five other circles. The quadrated portion introduces the concept of "four," which often is used numerically to represent wholeness. It is a "complete" number in the sense that there are four corners of the earth, four seasons in nature, or four basic elements in nature (fire, wind, water, and earth). Jung also identified four basic psychological functions—sensing, intuiting, thinking, and feeling—which we discuss later.

The mandala is a universal symbol appearing in many cultural, artistic, and physiological forms, emerging most often in Tibetan Buddhism. It also flourishes in Navaho sandpaintings. As you begin to seek it out, it surfaces in the architecture and symbols of many Western religious traditions. In nature, the mandala appears in the structure of a cell, in the form of the eye, in the sand dollar, and in the configuration of the solar system.

This use of the number four can be seen in some of the earliest medical practices. John Cule notes that the Greek idea about the cause of disease came from the humoral theory of the Sicilian

FIGURE 2-1

The Mandala As a Symbol for Soul

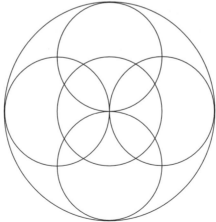

philosopher Empedocles (c. 500–430 B.C.),[6] who believed that everything was made from four elements: earth, air, fire, and water. This belief led to the idea that the physical states of health were determined by the balance of the four humors (or fluids): black bile, yellow bile, blood, and phlegm.

Soul As Web

Another profound, and even more relevant, image of soul is the web. Virtually everyone knows about the Internet World Wide Web, but here we refer to a living, not an electronic, connection.

In particular, the spiderweb (another example of the mandala in nature) serves as a metaphor for soul. The common notion views the spiderweb as an intricate wheel for catching food, but spiders construct webs for a variety of reasons—not only for sustenance but as a place to mate, raise their young, and rest. The spider creates a framework of radii, or spokes, in a certain pattern so that each radius will pull evenly on the web (figure 2-2). When the web is balanced, evenly tight all over, the spider senses even the slightest movement or vibration. A slight pull on one strand immediately affects the entire web. And the sum total dynamic or energy of the entire web is greater than the individual strands.

The web depicts another characteristic of soul, for soul too is greater than the sum of its parts. When a team of people, an organization, or a social unit connects to soul, the result is synergism (meaning 1 + 1 = 3). When we pull on one strand of the universal soul or the soul of an organization, for better or worse, we affect everything else because everything interrelates.

This interrelationship characteristic of soul calls into question the commonly held belief in American culture that everyone can do his or her own thing without regard for the consequences. It's the ethic of the self-made man (or woman) proclaiming a God-given right to personal freedom without considering its impact on other people and on social, economic, and environmental systems.

FIGURE 2-2

The Spiderweb As a Metaphor for Soul

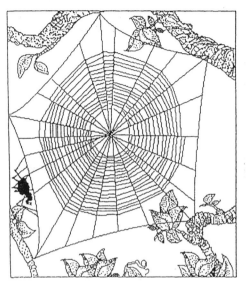

In any case, we can now formulate a metaphor for soul that we hope has meaning and impact in the twenty-first century. *Soul is mysterious, living, organic energy serving as a unifying, holistic web of connectedness throughout the universe.* We will use this metaphor from now on when we talk about soul.

The metaphor here is confirmed in contemporary microphysics and quantum physics. German physicist Max Planck coined the word *quantum* at the turn of the twentieth century, a Latin word meaning "how much." It was a way of showing energy as something paradoxically both smooth-flowing and ragged, predictable and unpredictable. Planck's observations, along with Einstein's theory of relativity, caused the sky to fall on the paradigm of the mechanical, deterministic universe.

In his foreword to *Space, Time and Medicine,* Capra suggests the following: "In twentieth-century physics, the universe is no longer perceived as a machine, made up of a multitude of separate objects, but appears as a harmonious indivisible whole; a web of dynamic relationships that include the human observer and his or her consciousness in an essential way."[7] So the paradigm shifts from machine to living web.

"A web of dynamic relationships" implies that any discussion of the nature of soul must be much more than an exercise of the mind. Soul primarily surfaces and is touched by *experience.* Soul is a fundamental encounter. To breathe is to experience soul, whether we are aware of it or not. Soul is something you sense, something that evokes feeling.

To enhance soul requires us to experience it in all that we do. There are many ways to encounter soul. We can connect with nature. We could also retreat to an art museum, find solitude in music, engage in memorable talk with family or friends, cook a meal at home, or work in a garden. However, to enhance soul in health care, we focus on four specific means (which we discuss in more depth later). They are:

- *Promoting individuality.* Carl Jung once remarked, "To know yourself is to know God." We could also affirm that to know yourself is to know soul. Soul naturally gravitates to activities that promote individual depth, meaning, value, and growth. Organizations encouraging individual expression and creativity enhance soul and are naturally more productive.
- *Advancing career satisfaction.* According to Moore, soul says, "Be good at what you are good at." Soul thrives on job satisfaction. Soul calls us to the work of our passion and deep pleasure.
- *Honoring diversity.* Being human involves the experience of differences and opposites. Soul flourishes in a work environment where diversity is honored. Soul also thrives on inner diversity.

• *Fostering community.* The presence of soul in business hinges on whether community is valued and nurtured. Synergism occurs when people experience a deep connection to others in work.

These four qualities of soul are not ordered in terms of priority or importance. If they were, we might begin with community. Unless we belong in a relationship with others and feel respected and cared for, it is almost impossible to progress and grow in maturity.

Soul, then, is like the chemistry drawing two people together into an intimate relationship. Even though difficult to explain, you know that a connecting energy, a magnetism, is present.

References

[1] Frederic Brussat and Mary Ann Brussat, *100 Ways to Keep Your Soul Alive, Living Deeply and Fully Every Day* (San Francisco: HarperSanFrancisco, 1994), p. xv.

[2] Marie Morgan and Mark Leavitt, "Recovering the Soul of Health Care," in *Rediscovering the Soul of Business, A Renaissance of Values,* eds. Bill De Foore and John Renesch (San Francisco: Sterling & Stone, 1995), p. 334.

[3] Thomas Moore, *Care of the Soul* (New York: HarperCollins, 1992).

[4] Lawrence Kushner, *Honey from the Rock: An Easy Introduction to Jewish Mysticism* (Woodstock, Vt.: Jewish Lights Publishing, 1994), p. 32.

[5] Tom Chappell, *The Soul of a Business* (New York: Bantam Books, 1993), p. xv.

[6] John Cule, "The History of Medicine," in *Medicine, A History of Healing,* ed. Roy Porter (New York: Barnes & Noble, 1997), p. 20.

[7] Fritjof Capra, foreword to *Space, Time and Medicine,* by Larry Dossey (Boulder, Colo.: Shambhala, 1982), p. x.

CHAPTER THREE

Soul—The Missing Dimension in Health Care

"What is the true business of healthcare? Is it the 'high-tech, high-touch' blend of dedicated caregivers and state-of-the-art technology that was promised in the 1980s? Or is healthcare purely a commodity—products and services that are bought and sold at the lowest price, on the spot market?"[1]

—Shari Mycek

*N*ot unlike other organizations and businesses, those in the health care industry continue to experience chaotic and ongoing transitions. Consider the rapid changes that have occurred just since 1995: a proliferation of mergers, alliances, joint ventures, and other newly evolving relationships. Keeping track of subsequent name changes and their not-for-profit or for-profit status has resulted in frustration rather like that found in the classic Abbott and Costello routine, "Who's on first?" This confusion is only compounded when old relationships break apart. The transitions not only affect larger institutions—individual hospitals and hospital systems—but also individual and group physician practices as well.

Much has already been said about the spiraling costs of medical care and the resulting debate over coverage. Little more then needs to be said other than to acknowledge the sky-rocketing level of anxiety that health care costs and payment-related issues create, not only for patients, but also for providers. Attempts to reduce costs while retaining quality of care have not been uniformly successful and have only added to the mounting distrust between the providers and receivers of health care services. The issue of cost has contributed greatly to the trauma resulting from ongoing transition.

Consider, too, a virtual alphabet soup of service providers ad infinitum: HMOs, PPOs, IPAs, HPOs, MSOs, PMOs. Health care professionals have a difficult enough time remembering what these acronyms stand for, let alone expecting the public to remember.

The consequences of such confusion remind one of the old TV show *Who Do You Trust?* The reality is that more and more people—patients, employees, and physicians—no longer trust the health care system. And increasing numbers of patients are losing trust in their physicians as well. John Cule states, "It is paradoxical that a decline in patient confidence in doctors in recent years has accompanied remarkable improvements in many therapies and in rates of curing previously fatal diseases."[2]

THE IMPACT OF CHANGE ON STAKEHOLDERS

The effects of the current bewildering health care environment have a significant impact on each of health care's audiences. And while a solution to the chaos is desirable, in fact it may be some time before improvement is seen. The key to a successful navigation of the rough seas of change is how organizations choose to respond to a chaotic environment and how they relate to each of their audiences. We believe that organizations lacking soul are less successful in managing transition. Loss of soul's connectedness directly relates to declining business profitability. To say it another way, soulful organizations are much more likely to survive chaos.

The Impact of Trauma on Physicians

The mounting level of frustration with a changing health care environment is taking its toll on physicians, who are struggling to find a meaningful balance between patient care and business expectations. New demands on physicians are leading to tragic consequences for many of them, resulting in the growing belief that the only help is to leave medicine altogether.

One physician verbalized this mounting frustration. She believes that for most physicians the decision to go to medical school stemmed from three basic motivations—the desire for autonomy, the desire to help others, and a belief in the possibility of making a good living. Today, however, she sees these motivators evaporating like dry ice.

Loss of Autonomy   Whether or not a physician is under contract, many physicians have lost their autonomy and freedom. One of the earlier strategies physicians developed to combat the growing irritation with managed care and increasing paperwork was merging their practices and joining groups with an administrative management structure. This arrangement anticipated taking business management out of the physicians' hands and enabling them to get back to the "practice of medicine." However, some of these integrated structures have failed to be the expected savior. A number of them have only added to the discontent, with the end result a loss of autonomy and a growing belief among physicians that they have become, as one former physician put it, an "interchangeable unit."

When a new multispecialty group was forming in a large metropolitan area, the group's managing partners, in their efforts to recruit doctors, made promises to alleviate some of the physicians' concerns about a changing environment. The group reassured the physicians that patients would be unaware that their physician had joined a large group. Benefits for their office employees would not decrease; in fact, in some instances they would be enhanced. Also, the corporate business organization pledged to be accountable to member physicians in a timely manner.

Once a physician joined, however, little effort was made to address his or her concerns. Policies changed, and promises once made went down the drain. Issues of significance to the physicians were ignored. Little concern was shown for either the physicians or their employees, all of whom perceived the group's tactics as a bait-and-switch con. Trust between the original physician members and the group's management vanished. The organization treated its members disrespectfully, and it ultimately went bankrupt.

Loss of Mission   The desire of physicians to help others—their vocational mission—has been compromised by outside pressures. One practitioner we interviewed sees the level of trust between patient and physician eroding, which she believes affects her real mission as a physician. "The patient/physician relationship was first adversely affected by lawyers. The fear of each [patient and physician] suing the other took away the atmosphere of trust. Today, it's the third-party payers that influence the relationship." She believes that now the payers, and even some institutions, have taken control away from the direct provider. Increasing paperwork and higher patient volume in shorter time periods are escalating the frustration of the entire office staff, which then reduces the pleasure of practicing medicine.

Another physician shared his mounting frustration. Pointing to a reproduction of one of Norman Rockwell's well-known pictures hanging in his office, he said, "That's why I went into medicine." The painting depicts a young boy standing in the examining room pulling down his slacks while intently looking at the physician's diploma. An older doctor is preparing the syringe. As only Norman Rockwell can, the picture captures the uncertain emotions of the young boy, yet conveys the feeling that somehow the doctor will do whatever is necessary to make things better.

According to this physician, however, today's medicine does not encourage a high level of time and involvement with patients. Because he works in a large clinic, patients move from one station to another as part of the diagnostic process: one station for blood pressure, another for weight, another for lab, and yet another for something else. As he likened the experience to an assembly line, the machine metaphor for medicine surfaced its ugly head.

"I almost left medicine because of this," he said, pointing to the clinic. But he reconsidered when offered the opportunity to direct a new specialized clinic with full authority to organize and direct it in the way he believes medicine should be delivered. Today, he is working hard to create a team that embodies the soul of medicine.

Decreasing Income Many physicians are reporting decreasing incomes. A number of reporting sources have suggested that the significant drop in income in 1994 attributed to managed care may have been stemmed. An increasing amount of compensation now is linked to incentives and bonuses.

Physicians increasingly believe they have few choices to remedy what they view as untenable situations. Attempts to regain control can lead to increasing collective bargaining, as evidenced by more physicians today looking to organized labor for support and advocacy. In May 1998, a large primary care medical group in the Northwest, consisting of nearly 230 physicians in a network of 46 primary care clinics, voted to join the United Salaried Physicians and Dentists Union. At that time, the union was said to represent the largest group of doctors in the private sector to organize. Reportedly, the group decided to join the union because of physician unhappiness over a lack of decision-making control, increasing patient loads, and unstable salaries. Physicians believe that where once their mission was to heal the patient, now the emphasis is on the bottom line. They see patients being called units and patient care being measured in productivity quotas.

The stress and disillusionment of health care today also results in early burnout and larger numbers of physicians choosing to leave medicine. One physician who left described first being aware of his professional burnout when he realized that he was more interested in moving a patient through the system than really listening to his patient's concerns.

Doctors are retiring earlier and many of them—experienced practitioners whom the medical field can ill afford to lose—are leaving in midcareer. Tom Curry of the Washington State Medical Association notes that the association keeps a database on retired members, and it appears that retirees are getting younger. He is concerned about losing physicians in their prime—their 50s. And a career specialist in the Dallas area reports that an increasing number of her clients are physicians leaving their practices.

What is happening with physicians affects new medical practitioners as well. A young medical student observed the current climate with its stresses: increased practice hours, reduced income, and career and family issues. He suggested that new physicians will have to decide the level of risk they are willing to take. In the past, new doctors acknowledged a level of physical risk, but today the risk goes much further.

The Impact of Trauma on Patients
Like a virulent virus, patient cynicism too is growing in this climate of physician stress. Many patients remain satisfied with their personal physician but express concern that the paperwork and time constraints now placed on doctors are beginning to erode their physician's ability to spend time with them. How many times have

we heard such comments as the following: "He [she] only spent a few minutes with me, but then sent a large bill"? Physicians who practice in larger groups or are employed by institutions are frequently "encouraged" to reduce their time with patients. One of the major complaints by physicians of the large, now unionized, primary care group mentioned earlier is the necessity to see more patients daily, which results in less time for each patient.

A recent survey of 6,100 physicians conducted by the University of Wisconsin Medical School emphasized the time dilemma.[3] Both male and female doctors in a variety of specialties indicated that they didn't have enough time to treat patients in the way they would like. Women physicians also reported seeing more patients with psychosocial problems, such as depression, anxiety, and eating disorders, that require more time.

Many observers believe that the time crunch is one of the issues fueling the public's growing interest in seeking alternative health care providers. It has been said that most physicians spend nine minutes with each patient and interrupt after only the first four seconds. Aside from an increasing interest in prevention and desire to manage their own health, more people believe that it is the alternative provider who will take the time to listen to their concerns. Acupuncturists reportedly spend an average of 90 minutes on a patient's first visit. One of the main reasons people change physicians is their dissatisfaction with how they are treated, whether the physician's inattention is the result of time constraints or not.

Actions Are Louder Than Words   The degree of patient suspicion can be observed in patients' reaction to a health care organization's mission statement. In an effort to convey the impression of heart and quality, a number of facilities use such words as *quality, excellence, caring, spirit,* and *heart.* Considerable amounts of money are often spent marketing these thematic phrases to the public, but patients don't always experience the action that goes with the words. One patient who was interviewed about satisfaction with health care said that such phrases in mission statements really sound like an ad agency wrote them. "Just because they say them doesn't make it necessarily so." It's not unusual to hear people discussing their experiences with hospitals—for example, "Today you have to look over your bills with a fine tooth comb to catch items billed for but not used."

When the soul of an organization diminishes, it can directly affect the trust between the patient and the physician or the organization. A high level of trust between doctor and patient contributes enormously to patient satisfaction. And there's evidence that better outcomes and greater compliance accompany increased patient satisfaction.

Conversely, a lack of trust encourages a lack of patient communication. During a focus session, a group of people were discussing their feelings about health care and their relationship with their physicians. A majority of the group stated that at one time or another they had seen, or continued to see on an ongoing basis, an alternative health care provider as well as their regular physician. Yet few believed they could tell their physician about this dual care because they were convinced they would be ridiculed by their doctor. This lack of trust can affect the efficacy of treatment when physicians are unaware of what other treatment is being used or what other products consumed.

In addition, patient trust erodes because of concern that physicians don't always order certain tests or prescribe treatments as a result of the pressure on them to minimize costs. Indeed, the media periodically report on patients being denied particular treatments on the assumption that denial of treatment is motivated by expense.

Patients are using the Internet with increasing frequency to learn about diseases and treatments and taking the information to their physician. Although the increasing number of well-informed patients who want to manage their health is a positive sign, it is also an indication of the erosion of unquestioning belief and trust in physicians.

The Impact of Trauma on Employees

We talked earlier about soul as an organic energy serving as a unifying, holistic web of connectedness and that this connectedness to the greater whole of healing draws many people into the world of health care. Employee morale is greatly affected by the degree of organizational soul. Organizations that undergo downsizing, reengineering, job redesign, or whatever the change is called, are particularly vulnerable to diminishing soul. One hospital administrator suggested that it is much easier to display soul in a financially healthy organization than one in financial turmoil, but organizational restructuring doesn't have to diminish an organization's soulfulness.

The High Cost of Diminished Soul In *Driving Fear Out of the Workplace,*[4] Ryan and Oestreich discuss the negative impact of fear on organizations. They recount the story of a senior administrator who reported how a recent restructuring had been sprung on the employees in spite of the organization's preaching "partnership and collegiality." The end result was an erosion of the emotional ties people had with the organization. The employees who didn't leave the organization worried when the next shoe would drop.

The costs associated with an employee's loss are significant. One such cost stems from replacing any employee who leaves. It has been estimated that in certain businesses it costs at least two times an employee's annual salary to replace him or her, especially when considering training time. If we were able to calculate the emotional expenses connected to the morale and performance of the remaining employees, the cost would be higher.

Another substantial cost, especially in this age of information technology, is the opportunity for unhappy employees to take with them an important client database or other business-related information. Being hired by a competitor could give the competitor a significant business advantage. As one secretary said, "If they fire me, I'm copying my disks."

Organizations that operate in an unsoulful manner are more likely to breed fear and an unwillingness by employees to take risks. The intangible costs of fear influence employees' feelings, relationships, quality of work, and productivity.

"Icy cold" described the atmosphere of a new, rapidly growing multispecialty group practice management office. "We versus them" best characterized the relationship between management and nonmanagerial staff. One senior manager periodically unleashed a scathing attack on employees whom she believed were not performing as she thought they should. Though she had no direct supervisory authority over these employees, their fear of her was unmistakable: in her presence their productivity decreased. One employee left the group as soon as she could find another job. No one dared complain to her boss, the CEO, from a recognition that key members of administration did not respect "lesser" employees. Such behaviors and lack of perceived mutual trust led to a pervasive unhappiness that was almost immediately felt by new employees. For them, the excitement of being part of a new organization soon evaporated, and the feeling of being connected to the group's overall goals was lost. Consequently, people began performing only the minimum requirements of their job; some secretly wished the group would fail. And it did fail!

In another situation, the director of a hospital medical records department told of working some years earlier in a psychiatric facility with a very closed administration. According to her, the administrator never spoke to lower-level employees except to place blame during times of lower inpatient admissions and consequently created an atmosphere of fear. Routines and procedures were regimented, but no attempt was made to communicate the administration's rationale. Working in this environment almost led our respondent to leave the health care field altogether.

Soul Provides the Glue during Transition   The senior administration of a medium-sized hospital facing the impact of a changing health care environment realized that changes were necessary for the hospital to remain competitive. While their financial picture was currently healthy, there was no guarantee that it would remain so. Although a reduction in the workforce was not foreseen, key management wanted to take proactive steps to prepare employees for the eventuality of future layoffs. Managers and then employees were kept fully informed of what was happening and the proactive stance the hospital was taking in a systematized, well-thought-out plan. While no one's job could be guaranteed safe, the hospital began a dialogue to address the major concerns of staff and to learn what employees expected of management in such a scenario. As a result of the dialogue, employees were promised that should downsizing occur, layoffs would not happen overnight and would not be a surprise. Employees then would be guaranteed jobs for a specified period to allow them time for transition to other jobs within the hospital or to find a position in another institution. And the hospital promised to use its contacts to find places for its laid-off employees.

Such a caring attitude went a long way in removing the fear that could have developed as employees observed those in other hospitals being laid off. It also encouraged employees to risk trying new responsibilities and to view their skills from the organization's perspective rather than from their usual sphere. The hospital successfully enhanced the feeling of trust and connectedness with its employees.

This particular hospital continues working hard to promote a relationship on which mutual trust and respect are built. One immediately senses this feeling of soul on entering the hospital and observes it in the delivery of patient care.

In another case, an older, large, well-respected hospital first experienced financial difficulties a few years ago at a time when there was a sense of connectedness among the staff and a feeling of being valued. Although a number of employees were laid off, the layoffs were performed in a caring and humane manner, including an acknowledgment of their contribution to the institution during their employment.

Some time later, continuing financial difficulties resulted in a reorganization. This time, however, the layoffs took place with little sensitivity. Even key administrative staff were not exempt. In fact, one of the administrators who had orchestrated the former staff reduction so tastefully found herself without a job. She reportedly was simply told in the morning that her job was gone and to have her office cleaned out by the end of the afternoon. Here we witness two very different ways of handling difficult situations— one an example of a soulful approach and the latter devoid of soulful respect; the latter approach led a physician to describe the hospital as now lacking in soul.

THE IMPACT OF SOUL ON THE BOTTOM LINE

The presence of soul, or its apparent absence, can certainly affect the bottom line of an organization. It affects not only internal stakeholders but external customers as well. We look below at how soul influences patient satisfaction and the cost of attracting and keeping patients. The importance of patient satisfaction cannot be overstated or overestimated. Emphasis on patients was underscored in fact by *Modern Healthcare*'s designation of 1998 as the Year of the Patient.

Patient Satisfaction

Earlier we suggested that patient discontent results in patients' diminishing trust in physicians and the health care delivery system in general. We talked about the patient-physician relationship, but spent less time on how frontline employees contribute to the success or failure of an organization's business. As one professor pointed out, patient-physician interaction in a hospital counts for only a small portion of a patient's experience. The attitudes of the staff that provides the bulk of direct patient contact, however, greatly affect patient satisfaction. As one midlevel hospital manager said, "Unhappy employees don't have to say anything [to affect patient satisfaction]. Patients can see their body language and feel their attitudes."

Although patients are becoming more sophisticated and knowledgeable about treatment options, they still can't evaluate the clinical or technical expertise of institutions or practitioners. What they do know is how they are treated. They know when people listen to them, respond in a timely manner, treat them with respect, and help them navigate the difficult waters of "organizationalese." Silence is not an attribute of the unhappy patient. Patients who haven't had their expectations met or have had a poor experience will tell a minimum of at least 10 others about their experience, and the listeners will in turn pass the news along, most probably altered. Dissatisfied patients may try once again, particularly if they complained and were listened to, or they may refuse ever to return. And no matter their choice, they can influence others.

It's been said there are only three ways of obtaining patients: keep current patients, reactivate inactive patients, or attract new patients. By far, the cheapest method is keeping current patients. Many practices and clinics are unaware of the reason why some of their patients don't return. When one fairly busy OB/GYN practice noticed that a number of its patients were leaving the practice and not returning for ongoing care, no effort was made to discover the reason. The physicians blamed managed care, suggesting that women didn't have a choice when their provider plans changed. The declining patient base affected admissions to the physicians' primary hospital, so the hospital requested outside help to learn the reason for the changing patient pattern. A discussion with the physicians' nurses, along with further investigation, revealed that increasing numbers of patients not only were unhappy with the practice but also expressed dissatisfaction with the hospital. And their discontent had little to do with clinical expertise.

In another example, a former patient told of lying in a very cold hospital room, but frequent complaints of being cold went unheeded. At one point, the patient reported that he was told to remain calm because it takes time for a room to warm up. Unwisely, this patient checked himself out of the hospital because of the staff's attitude. Even if extreme, this example points out the importance of patient dissatisfaction.

When a young couple delivered their first child in a small hospital, the new mother (whom we shall call Sarah) shared a semiprivate room with a woman who received multiple groups of visitors. At one point the room was so full that there was no place for Sarah's husband and one visitor to sit. Although the couple complained, the nurses appeared either unable or unwilling to enforce the hospital's rules. Sarah couldn't get sufficient rest or sleep that night because of the noise, so she requested an early discharge. She shared this story many times over with friends and relatives. As she said, "It's no wonder the other [competitor] hospital is attracting away more patients."

The High Cost of Marketing

Consider, too, the high cost of attracting new patients. The marketing and advertising budgets of hospitals and health care systems are increasing rapidly. In fact, according to an Opinion Research Corporation International survey, the average hospital marketing budget increased 5 percent in 1997, from $467,400 a year earlier to $492,000. The average hospital advertising budget jumped 32 percent from $195,100 in 1996 to $257,800 in 1997.[5]

Larger budgets may be a reflection of bigger systems that are faced with the continuous need to clarify to their constituents the frequent mergers, affiliations, and name and access changes. However, even smaller organizations believe they must increase their marketing efforts if they are to remain competitive. In both groups, marketing and advertising budgets are believed critical in keeping and/or adding to their patient base.

Consider the high cost of a direct mail campaign designed to position a new service. The goals may not only include building awareness but also gaining an immediate trial of the service. But if patients who respond are met by staff who are less than welcoming, if patients perceive themselves as merely an interruption to the staff, and if patients' expectations are not met, the likelihood of their trying the service again is slim.

Evidence of the importance of patient satisfaction can be seen by an increasing number of special patient satisfaction programs implemented in health care organizations. The programs may be designated with acronyms that denote "heart" or caring and are designed to sensitize employees to the importance of satisfied patients. Or following in the footsteps of a number of corporate businesses, health care organizations have implemented service excellence programs. Although these efforts are to be applauded, early positive results are frequently not maintained. In many instances, employees' telephone demeanor, monitored response time to a patient's call light, and so on are simply remote, taught behaviors. Reminders or incentives are required for internalization. We suggest that organizations first pay attention to soul and create an atmosphere of respect that honors individuality, diversity, career satisfaction, and community. Creating such an atmosphere prepares the ground for the seeds of patient satisfaction programs to take root and spread.

A patient's wife, for example, was talking about the couple's experience in a hospital some miles from where they lived. "You know," she said, "it was wonderful. Every time we went [there], everyone, including the groundskeeper, wondered how he [her husband] was doing!" Obviously, she was impressed with the genuine caring of someone whose responsibility was not patient care. She loved telling the story. Clearly, there was a connectedness to the overall mission of the hospital that transcended specific job responsibilities.

Not only do satisfied patients refer others to health care providers—so do employees of the providers. A bank staff member's discontent, although in an entirely different setting, nonetheless makes the point: "The bank has changed its relationship to its employees. Loyalty, trust, and the family sense are gone. It's them and us—they would lay you off tomorrow if it fit a corporate interest. This certainly has reduced loyalty in return. I wouldn't recommend this bank to a friend."[6] Employee connectedness to the overall mission is especially important in health care organizations.

In a major regional medical center, department managers operated with respect for one another. Respect splashed over to external customers as well, including the vendors with whom the managers dealt. When one department director resigned, she was replaced by an individual who treated others, including her vendors, with contempt. She seldom returned phone calls, kept people waiting, and made it clear that her duties were of greater importance than others. As a result, some of the vendors, who had typically offered extra discounts or went out of their way to service the center, became less accommodating. Some began demanding payment COD or charging for project estimates. The moral of this story is that vendors and other colleagues are just as much an organization's potential partners, patients, or referral sources as are those to whom the organization regularly markets.

References

[1] Shari Mycek, "Leadership for a Healthy 21st Century," *Healthcare Forum Journal* (July/August, 1998): 26.

[2] John Cule, "The History of Medicine," in *Medicine, A History of Healing,* ed. Roy Porter (New York: Barnes & Noble, 1997), p. 15.

[3] Carol Smith, "Doctors Burn Out Early and Some Call It Quits," *Seattle Post-Intelligencer* (May 26, 1998), pp. A1–A5.

[4] Kathleen D. Ryan and Daniel K. Oestreich, *Driving Fear Out of the Workplace* (San Francisco: Jossey-Bass, 1991), p. 229.

[5] Deanna Bellandi, "Big Ad Bucks," *Modern Healthcare* (April 6, 1998): 82.

[6] Ryan and Oestreich, *Driving Fear Out of the Workplace,* p. 56.

CHAPTER FOUR

Paradigm Shift

*"God gives you this gift of healing;
it's up to you to use it well."*

—Bruce Francis, MD, Seattle

$\mathcal{F}$or more than 200 years we have used a machine as the metaphor for how we see the world. We talk about people being cogs in the wheel of business and industry. We say, "A good business is run like a well-oiled machine." Many people use the same metaphor to describe health care, and some physicians even view the human body as a machine. Perceiving the world in this light perpetuates a particular belief system, which then dictates our actions and forms the basis of the way we approach others in our organization and the patients with whom we have contact.

A NEW METAPHOR

$\mathcal{T}$oday we are moving into a new era—from the industrial age to the information age. Such a shift requires us to describe things differently and to change our belief system about how the world operates. The machine metaphor no longer works. Earlier, we suggested a new metaphor for health care that we believe offers a meaning and impact in the twenty-first century. With our declaration that

> *"I know that for every door that closes, another door opens. But, man! Those hallways are a bitch!"*
>
> —T-shirt motto
>
>

soul is mysterious, living, organic energy serving as a unifying, holistic web of connectedness throughout the universe, the emphasis shifts from the idea of machine to one of a living, invisible web of interconnectedness. This way of looking at the universe is particularly meaningful to health care—the tapestry of caring and compassion places people ahead of machines.

Consider the interconnectedness of cyberspace and the proliferation of information systems that form a network of patient information and outcome data. Partnering and crucial alliances become strategies. Observe the health care systems that have created strategic alliances with other complementary industries such as pharmaceutical companies and suppliers. Partnering is not machinelike. Unlike machines where cogs and parts can be replaced with little impact on the whole, we cannot replace people without notice. Like the spiderweb illustration used earlier, change, for better or worse, results in a pull on the organization.

HEALTH CARE'S MISSION IN HISTORY

*W*e suggested earlier that soul is deeply connected to the essence of health care's core healing mission or calling. Some of the elements of this link can be traced to early times; our medical history is rich with references to healing. Our purpose here is not to document a history of health care, but rather to note briefly the diverse beginnings of the medicine we know today. It is the connection to the whole that bears note.

The varied history of the different types of early healing is reviewed in *Medicine, A History of Healing*.[1] There is written evidence of Egyptian medicine in ancient texts from 10,000 to 2000 B.C. Also during this period of history, herbal medicines were used in Mesopotamia and China; the legendary emperor Shen Nong (3494 B.C.) discovered herbal medicine. There is evidence of the medicinal use of herbs by Egyptians and the use of needles and trephination in the Stone Age. From the extraordinarily detailed recordkeeping of the ancient Chinese, we know Chinese acupuncture is among the oldest and most effective and successful therapies.[2]

Two of the earliest recorded healers were the Yellow Emperor, legendary founder of Chinese medicine (2698–2598 B.C.), and Imhotep in Egypt, c. 2980 B.C. The practice of medicine was referred to as "noble" in Homer's *Iliad*.[3]

When tribal medicine was replaced by civilized and rational curiosity about the cause of illness, true medical science in the West began. One of the most well known of the early healers was Hippocrates of Kos (460–377 B.C.).[4] He based his practice on careful bedside observation and understood the importance of keeping records of case histories. Considered the "father of Western medicine," Hippocrates developed a set of ethical standards for the medical profession, and his teachings influenced the ethical relationship of doctor to patient. He inspired the Hippocratic oath (which is no longer universally recited by graduating physicians).

Over the years, the progression of Western medicine retreated from a belief in the inner connectedness of the mind, body, and spirit to one that focuses more on the repair of the body. Yet true soulful healing as a mission leads us in a different direction. In appealing for a new medicine, Gordon states that "it [new medicine] insists, as did the tribal shamans who were our first healers, that the work, the 'profession' of those who 'provide' health care, is itself a spiritual path."[5]

Morgan and Leavitt look at the historical progression in this way:

I'm reminded of a 16th Century history, when scientists were trying to define a different reality than the church's worldview.
Clearly it was a needed correction at the time, but the polarization
between spirit and "pure" objectivity has outlived its usefulness. I
also find it amusing that cultures all over the world have had their
shamans, their gifted healers, yet we in our Western European tradition assume there would be no such healers amongst us. I find it
quite plausible that our physicians, nurses, and, yes, other "alternative" practitioners, might also be endowed with healing instincts,
healing gifts. I know many health care providers who feel a very
deep sense of calling but rarely talk about it. Physicians and other
mainstream caregivers are not currently free—or encouraged—to
deal with people in wise, holistic ways.[6]

The good news is that technology has become more sophisticated, enabling physicians and other healers to diagnose and treat
illnesses that heretofore were considered fatal. The downside is the
temptation to increase dependency on machines as a substitute for
personal diagnostic skills. One physician who was interviewed
bemoaned this loss when he suggested that we have given our pro-
fessionalism over to machines. "Technology has made us a society
where the doctor-patient relationship has been affected by the
machine. In the past it was the skills of the physician that made diagnosis possible." One professor of medical history and ethics agrees,
believing that health care's mission has been compromised because
we have become highly technical. He worries that in the future doctors will be "corporatized." They will seldom observe, nor will they
practice, medicine as it was practiced before the emphasis on technology. No one advocates the elimination of technology. Rather, its
benefits should be applied as an adjunct tool.

If we are to return to health care's original mission, we must
change our belief system. No longer can we afford to equate healing
and compassion with a machinelike delivery of care. Optimum care

requires us to embrace the interrelatedness of those who have responsibility for the delivery of care.

IMPLICATIONS FOR WORK OF A NEW METAPHOR

*C*hanging the machine metaphor will require a significant shift in the way in which we look at all aspects of our health care delivery process. In figure 4-1, we see the paradigmatic shift in the way we approach work. The old paradigm emerged from the seventeenth century perceptions of Francis Bacon, Rene Descartes, and Isaac Newton, in which the universe is objectified and quantified. As a result, people and their jobs tend to be viewed for the most part as boring and machinelike. Work tends to be broken up into piecemeal tasks for the sake of greater productivity. People work mainly for money, not for self-satisfaction.

With the new paradigm, as perceived by theoretical physicists, the world cannot be seen as a system of independent parts like billiard balls glancing off each other. The universe becomes a single system unified and interrelated like a single living cell. In such a cosmos there is beauty, intricate ordering, and purposefulness. In our work we

> *"Doctors are not mechanics, responsible simply for repairing broken parts. We shouldn't act that way, or if we want to, we should do the perfectly honorable work of tending to machines. The work we've chosen, the promise our position holds out to suffering people, is different. We are there to be present for and serve people with real and complex lives and with thoughts and feelings about every aspect of those lives. . . . If we say we want to create a healing partnership with them, [our patients], they will likely be surprised and very pleased."[7]*
>
> —James S. Gordon
>
>

participate in an evolving and creative process. Each job, no matter how small, holds meaning for the individual worker and brings at least an element of satisfaction. Each task contributes to the whole.

What are the implications of such a substitution of the metaphor for work in health care? Referring to the model in figure 4-1, we look at a few health care professions and suggest how a belief system can affect the work behavior in each.

FIGURE 4-1

Paradigms and Their Implications for Work

Old Paradigm	Implications for Work	New Paradigm	Implications for Work
The world is a machine.	*People are treated like machines at work. They have no humanity.*	The world is an organism. Everything is alive and growing.	*Work springs from an inner, hidden "seed" or creativity. It is involved in growth and the creative process.*
The universe and its bodies are inanimate and without purpose.	*Work is drudgery, a matter of manipulation, and has no intrinsic reward.*	The universe and its bodies operate within "fields" or places of attraction.	*Work is connected to that which attracts and interests a person and to that which a person enjoys.*
All matter is primarily inert.	*Work is necessarily boring, without surprise or spontaneity.*	Atoms are structures of activity located in fields of energy and self-organizing systems.	*To work is to rearrange, invent, and make possible, and is full of surprise and wonder.*

Adapted from Matthew Fox, *The Reinvention of Work* (San Francisco: HarperCollins, 1994), and Joseph Jaworski, *Synchronicity, The Inner Path of Leadership* (San Francisco: Berrett-Koehler Publishers, 1996).

Physicians

Under the old work paradigm, many physicians believed they had the sole responsibility for the diagnosis, cure, and care of their patients' health. This belief creates an aura of infallibility—doctors as godlike in their knowledge and ability—and perpetuates a conviction by patients that their doctors are quick to write a prescription for everything. If there is no drug to fix it, then it can't be fixed. Such beliefs place a heavy burden of responsibility on the physician, creating a level of expectation that cannot be met.

> *"Medicine may be largely a body of knowledge, but healing is a personal skill."*[8]
>
> —Roy Porter

The new paradigm, however, encourages partnership between patient and physician. Patients are encouraged to take responsibility for the management of their health. Technology is not the be-all and end-all but only one piece of the diagnostic or treatment puzzle. Physicians are seen as skilled and knowledgeable but also as human. Doctors are free to become teachers. To suggest such a partnership between patients and physicians is not only enormously freeing but also fosters an atmosphere of mutual trust and respect. Each has a responsibility in the patient's overall health and well-being.

On the other hand, the lack of a patient-physician partnership impedes communication. Patients frequently forget some of the items they wish to discuss, or they feel pressured to talk fast—to get it all in before the doctor leaves the room. Already possibly anxious about their visit, such communication concerns can lead to situationally raised blood pressure and respiration. Conversely, a feeling of partnership lends itself to shared communication—concern and knowledge, question and answer, teacher and student. Time is perceived as less of a constraint.

Senior Management

Under the old paradigm, members of senior management are frequently selected because of their skills in "fixing" a particular problem, department, or organization. In fact, many CEOs or other top administrators have employment contracts that include a "golden parachute" clause, which encourages the belief that termination will occur when an executive outlives his or her usefulness. Consider the implications of such a belief system. There is no necessity to create an atmosphere of trust or shared responsibility. Truly, "the buck stops here": the assignment of ultimate responsibility drives organizational direction and problem solving. A revolving door in management does not create a soulful work attitude.

"My responsibility is to help people to discover for themselves what is best for them. I'm there to share my knowledge and whatever wisdom I may have, and to help them understand their lives and explore their options. . . . I see myself primarily as a healer and guide. The derivation of the word doctor *from the Latin* docere—'to teach'—*suits me and confirms me in this role."*[9]

—James S. Gordon

Information and problem solving are directed downward under the old paradigm. Employees are treated as a negative asset. In times of financial difficulty, employee-related costs are frequently the first to be axed. Some managers are even known for their tactics of "slash and burn" as a way of creating financial viability and improved profits. Senior administration appears closed and information is shared only on a need-to-know basis. Contact with lower-level employees occurs primarily when problems arise, and blame comes before problem solving. There is a strong perception of "we versus them."

Planning and business development may be purely a function of key management without an understanding of how projects will affect the individuals chiefly responsible for implementation. In some organizations, marketing directors may be seen only as those who implement the ideas spawned by senior management. The new paradigm suggests an atmosphere of shared responsibility. Management and frontline employees share responsibility equally for the organization's success. Employees are acknowledged for their contributions. Information and suggestions for improvement are shared, and management is a two-way process. Employees are seen as critical to the success of the organization and, as such, information is routinely and systematically shared with everyone. Problem solving is directed to those employees who, on a day-to-day basis, are best qualified to fix the problem. People who make it happen have input into solutions.

The medical records director of a small hospital tells the story of an apparently insoluble problem. The clinical nursing directors were given the responsibility of making certain that consistent charting was done by following a specific medical procedure. Numerous meetings were held with the nurses responsible for compliance. Compliance improved immediately following directives and meetings; however, it didn't last. After two years, it was decided to assign the project to all of the nurses and technicians involved in the procedure to see whether a new system for documentation could be developed. Once the frontline employees worked together, a simple solution emerged; the rate of compliance increased and remained high. The solution was already there, but no one had thought to ask the employees who were responsible for the service. "People want to feel that they have control over their jobs. It's the little things that make employees leave."

In the soulful organization, all employees are equally important. One CEO of a large medical center was known for respecting his employees, and he fostered this respect in others. He knew the names of the housekeepers just as well as he did the names of his department directors. It was not unusual for him to talk with the cooks in the kitchen while keeping waiting a physician who had dropped by to see him. The value he placed on others made a difference in how people saw their roles in the organization.

In times of financial difficulty, employees share in planning for cost-saving measures. Attention is paid to the process of managing transition before reorganization, mergers, or alliances take place. Any necessary layoffs are done in humane and respectful ways.

Marketing/PR Professionals
Under the old paradigm, the temptation is to view marketing and planning in a way that supports particular strategies or organizational objectives. Marketing activities may represent short-term objectives that are detached from the overall picture of the organization. Corporate alliances, mergers, or other partnerships may be viewed only from the perspective of profitability and increased market share; they may not be considered in light of whether such decisions compromise the organization's mission and values. New programs or services may be dictated without regard to their impact on current programs, staffing levels, or employee responsibilities. When this happens, individuals responsible for the implementation of such programs become less interested in overall business profitability and more focused on how "doable" their added responsibilities will be. Potentially, such a scenario can adversely affect patient satisfaction.

The new paradigm perpetuates joint responsibility for the group's success. Marketing objectives appear less contrived, becoming a natural extension of the organization's operation. Department heads and personnel are consulted and listened to as a part of the strategic planning process. Business strategies are integrated and support the overall mission of the group. Marketing is not an isolated activity.

A large medical center in the West developed a new children's activity program as one element in its strategy to build physician referrals and to increase its pediatric patient census. An interdepartmental task group was developed to create one of the program's core components. Because this was a group effort, the enthusiasm, excitement, and ownership felt by the team permeated the end product. Throughout the ensuing years, the core team felt personal responsibility for the program's success in all of the additional activities that the program generated. It became one of the most documented successes for the medical center's marketing efforts.

Nursing and Other Care/Ancillary Services

In most health care settings, nursing professionals stand as the core component of clinical care. They are the staff most responsible for the ongoing treatment and care of their patients, but they don't carry out their tasks in a vacuum. They must function as a team with other caregivers and support service personnel. Consider organizations in which interconnectedness of units or areas is not considered central to operations. In such a scenario, each area functions as an independent cog or business center. Such a disconnection encourages feelings of territorialism. Office and staffing resources are seen as limited and to be protected at any cost.

In addition, it is relatively easy with a lack of interconnectedness to shift employees without consideration of the ramifications. For many years, a large, well-known institution was recognized for the level of its medical care. Previously identified as a soulful organization, its image changed as a result of employee cuts. In an effort to reduce employee costs and benefits, long-term staff nurses were systematically let go and replaced by pool or agency nurses. Such actions reflected negatively on the quality of care, on physician and patient satisfaction, and on issues of risk management, and would not have happened under the new paradigm, which fosters a feeling of belonging to the same team. Nursing and other departments function as one team and share responsibility in patient care. The director of nursing in one hospital reported that when she walked into the hospital one morning and spoke to one of the housekeepers, the housekeeper was taken aback and said, "You are the first nurse who ever talked to me."

Health care is filled with many such examples that illustrate the relationship of work to our belief systems, the paradigm we embrace. Admittedly, we have focused here primarily on hospital settings, but work behaviors easily translate to other positions within different health care venues (discussed in chapter 9). The degree to which organizations and their employees function as an integrated unit contributes to a ripple effect throughout the organization. Having set the stage for this paradigm shift, we will explore ways in which organizations can enhance their soulfulness.

References

[1] Roy Porter, ed., *Medicine, A History of Healing* (New York: Barnes & Noble, 1997), p. 8.

[2] John Cule, "The History of Medicine," in *Medicine, A History of Healing,* ed. Roy Porter (New York: Barnes & Noble, 1997), p. 19.

[3] Porter, *Medicine,* p. 8.

[4] Cule, "History," p. 20.

[5] James S. Gordon, *Manifesto for a New Medicine, Your Guide to Healing Partnerships and the Wise Use of Alternative Therapies* (New York: Addison-Wesley, 1996), p. 18.

[6] Marie Morgan and Mark Leavitt, "Recovering the Soul of Health Care," in *Rediscovering the Soul of Business, A Renaissance of Values,* eds. Bill De Foore and John Renesch (San Francisco: Sterling & Stone, 1995), p. 333.

[7] Gordon, *Manifesto,* p. 247.

[8] Porter, *Medicine,* p. 7.

[9] Gordon, *Manifesto,* p. 87.

CHAPTER FIVE

Soul and Individuality

*"A soulful personality is complicated,
multifaceted, and shaped by both pain and
pleasure, success and failure. Life lived soulfully
is not without its moments of darkness and
periods of foolishness. Dropping the salvational
fantasy frees us up to the possibility of self-
knowledge and self-acceptance, which are the
very foundation of soul."* [1]

—Thomas Moore

*J*ohn walks into the doctor's office, ready for his annual physical.
The interior waiting room offers little to suggest a warm "hello."
Aging, almost unnoticeable pictures hang as if desperately clinging
to worn-out, dirty beige painted walls. No one smiles at John, not
even the receptionist behind the sliding, frosted window. Because
this is his first visit, he completes the personal information and
medical history form.

After a half-hour or so wait, a nurse ushers him into a small
enclosed cubicle, painted white, and he sits on the edge of the
paper-covered examining table. Another 20 minutes pass, more
than sufficient time to ponder the nature and meaning of an
anatomical chart on the wall.

Finally the doctor arrives and John senses his rush to fill a daily quota of consultations. After a few casual introductory remarks, the examination begins. John recites the usual litany of "nos" to questions concerning the status of his anatomy. Reflexes are challenged. The ears, eyes, nose, throat, and heart are checked. His body is prepared for a prostate gland review. John's prescriptions are filled and off he goes for the customary draining of fluids. As he leaves the office, John wonders whether the doctor would ever like to know something about his "story" as well as his physical being.

Like John, most of us yearn to share our personal stories. It is perhaps the easiest and most profound way of connecting with others and to soul. In this chapter, we look at the relationship between storytelling and individuality, the process of becoming conscious individuals and identifying with what Carl Jung called the "shadow," and the difference between codependence and differentiation.

STORYTELLING AND INDIVIDUALITY

In earlier times, explorers visiting African bushmen tribes reported having difficulty establishing meaningful relationships at first. The tribespeople were reluctant to share their personal and tribal stories because they believed that the soul literally resides in their stories. To tell a story meant that part of one's soul was being released to the listener.

Many of our personal stories reflect our humanity and earthiness; sharing them helps connect us to soul. Even some of the simple events of an ordinary day become subjects for recital; some of them make us laugh at ourselves or others because they reveal our foolishness and failures.

Storytelling serves as a relatively safe way to enhance soul and individuality because to be alive is to have a unique story. No two people have exactly the same story. Indeed, two people may experience the same event, but they often end up describing it in remarkably different ways, which is why, during a medical emergency, caregivers seek as much information and as many accounts of the situation as possible.

Humans are people who think and talk in stories because stories convey deeply felt meaning, as if someone else's story could have been yours as well. Storytelling often inspires passion and empathy. When someone tells about losing a set of car keys at a critical moment, we feel sorry for that person. Or when a person reports an unexpected and delightful surprise, we share in the delight.

One physician lamented the lack of opportunity for hearing more of his patient's stories. In discussing this loss of relationship, he noted that even though he spends time with his patients, he never really learns all their stories—who they really are in their community. When he sees them, they present him with a story of illness.

"You know," he said, "I often go to the funerals of my patients. When I hear the eulogies about who they were, what they cared for, and what they have done, I feel sad that I did not know them in that way."

> *"Everybody has a story. When I was a child, people sat around kitchen tables and told their stories. We don't do that so much anymore. Sitting around the table telling stories is not just a way of passing time. It is the way the wisdom gets passed along. The stuff that helps us to live a life worth remembering. Despite the awesome powers of technology, many of us still do not live very well. We may need to listen to each other's stories once again."[2]*
>
> —Rachel Naomi Remen
>
>

Joseph Campbell was regarded as a man with a thousand stories. For many, he restored the power of myth—fables particularly connecting us to soul. Many people misuse the word *myth,* falsely

assuming that because the story may not actually have happened, it
carries little significance. Whether fact or fantasy, the key issue of a
myth lies in its meaning. Does the story generate emotion? Does it
activate the imagination? Does it harmonize body and mind with
soul?

Stories also evoke self-understanding and creativity, and sometimes they bring light to the paths we travel in life. As we shall see
later, significant work experiences throughout one's life often
reveal patterns in key skills and professional orientation.

One of us (Jim, the coauthor of this book) has been meeting
weekly with a support group of men, who early on decided to
begin by sharing life stories in segments according to age. For
example, members of the group would reflect on significant
events that happened when they were 10 to 15 years old.
One person might speak about working at a part-time job in
order to purchase a bicycle and another about an unfortunate
relocation to a new town, which sparks the memory of others in
the group who have had a similar experience. A deepening sense of
intimacy occurs through this storytelling.

> "Without storytelling, it
> would be difficult to
> imagine how a people or
> an organization could pass
> on collective wisdom,
> teach new members about
> how to behave and what it
> means to belong, and
> convey the knowledge
> needed to survive in the
> natural or corporate world.[3]
>
> —Richard Stone

In *The Soul of a Business,* Chappell reminds us that in an organization, "my" story conjoins with "our" story. Like individuals,
organizations acquire a history and therefore have stories to tell.
"The essence of any company—its identity," says Chappell, "is
found in its beliefs, its values and its stories."[4] To propagate such
stories throughout the organization and particularly to newcomers

serves to enhance the soul of the association. Without the telling and retelling of corporate tales and anecdotes, human effort can waffle in almost meaningless production.

One physician related an incident in which a clinical practice experienced new leadership resulting from a reorganization. Sadly, whenever staff wanted to talk about stories in either their previous organization or their current one, management effectively squashed such attempts. The inability to recognize the importance of the human story resulted in a sterile and unfeeling group.

Also, there is an essential distinction between the open story and the closed story. Like the history of humankind, an open-ended story continues to unfold. Like an extinct culture or species, the closed story is finished. The former captivates us with its possibilities, such as the introduction of a new technology, product line, or customer service opportunity. It sparks imagination and enthusiasm for the tasks ahead. In contrast, the closed story often evokes the image of an organization that has lost its vitality. It may have gone beyond the prime of success and is experiencing decay, such as a hospital or health care organization serving a declining patient population. Its structure, policies, and values have become calcified, bureaucratic, and rigid. Such an organization remains anchored to the past and may become a prime candidate for acquisition, reorganization, or reengineering.

Enhancing Storytelling in the Organization
A few of the many ways to propagate stories in an enterprise are the following:

- Include organizational history in the organization's policies and procedures manual. Like other material, this history can be updated periodically.
- Assign storytelling responsibilities to specific individuals and especially to those who routinely interface with employees,

such as trainers or other human resources personnel. In fact, one CEO stated he assigned the position of storyteller to a specific trainer.

- Involve as many employees as possible in the creation of a vision or mission statement, then routinely publish examples of how it is being achieved.
- Publish individual and group human interest stories in the internal publication or through newsletters. (See chapter 9 for an excellent example of storytelling.)
- Routinely practice a simple, organizational development technique called appreciative inquiry (AI) that surveys work groups to inquire about things that are going well. AI builds on successes and systems that are functioning soundly and then seeks to promote those activities even further in the organization. (See chapter 8 for more information about AI.)
- Plan events to celebrate milestones. Encourage gatherings before or after work and during coffee breaks and lunch hours. Whenever possible, mix groups by including diverse disciplines and hierarchical blend.

THE INDIVIDUATION PROCESS

According to Thomas Moore, care of the soul begins by continually exploring and developing a keen sense of who we are as individuals. It involves a lifelong inquiry and journey. Carl Jung largely broke away from his pioneering association with Sigmund Freud over individuation. Freud, whose training was in biology and medicine, developed convincing arguments that biological and sexual instincts largely motivate human behavior. In part, Jung rejected this thesis, maintaining that we have an even stronger will to live, to grow, and to move toward a state of completion that he called the individuation process. We might say that Freud was a reductionist, reducing behavior to its biological origins, and Jung an expansionist, seeing in people a desire to be whole.

The overriding goal of Jungian analysis is assisting people to become individuals. It means not only being shaped and influenced by one's environment but being one's own person with one's own ideas, history, and unique experiences. To individuate means developing one's own identity apart from how we have been shaped by others.

> *"One always learns one's mystery at the price of one's innocence."*
>
> —Robertson Davies,
> *Fifth Business*
>
>

Jung's *Modern Man in Search of a Soul* focuses on the individuation process. It describes the lifelong journey of becoming conscious of who we are and characterizes the voyage as one toward enlightenment and self-actualization, "seeing" one's actual self in its many dimensions.

Figure 5-1 illustrates the complexity of a human being. Who we are constitutes many factors, including nationality, sexuality, vocation, religion, education, family of origin, physical makeup, age, and level of maturity; but lurking deep within each of us is a vast unknown. In reality, this vast unknown encompasses much more of who we are than the 30 percent depicted in the diagram; more than 90 percent of our totality actually resides in the unknown. What we consciously know about ourselves is like an island in the ocean or like a gigantic dark cave with many deep rooms where light from a small torch illuminates all we can see and comprehend.

In *Boundaries of the Soul,* June Singer reports that during her doctoral examination, she was asked to describe individuation as if she were talking to a street sweeper while waiting for the bus.[5] She answered by picturing a sailboat on a lake being blown by the wind; wind is felt and experienced but not controlled, although the wind must be observed carefully and understood for a sailor to make progress. Life movement and growth toward knowing oneself are comparable to adjusting the sails and direction of a boat to the nuances of the wind, a never-ending process.

FIGURE 5-1

Human Complexity

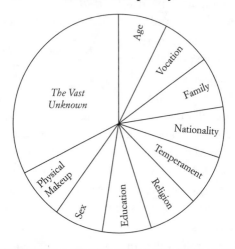

EXPLORING YOUR UNKNOWN

*T*here are many ways to explore your vast inner unknown:

- Lifelong learning, either on the job or in the classroom, certainly expands self-awareness. Often during the beginning of a workshop, we ask participants to report their years of paid work experience. Individual years are tallied to arrive at a composite figure for the group. Depending on the size of the group, the figure reaches high into the hundreds. This exercise illustrates the group resources and knowledge available to be tapped during the learning process.

- Receiving and processing feedback from others are ways to expand self-understanding. Others often see elements of personality that remain hidden from ourselves.

• Many people keep a journal, recording thoughts, feelings, and images related to life events. One popular technique involves engaging in a dialogue with an image or aspect of oneself and recording whatever comes to mind, thus helping to bring to the surface buried information and insights.

• Working with one's dreams is an excellent pathway to one's inner world. Every element in a dream portrays some part of the psyche. Although quite helpful, it is not essential to visit an analyst to understand the messages of dreams. Jim spent two and one-half years in analysis with two different professionals. Occasionally, he accused them of engaging in four or more years of training in order to ask the question, "What does the dream mean to you?" We can ask that of ourselves and conduct word associations with aspects of our dreams.

• Some schools of thought suggest that everything we need to know about ourselves we already know. The answers to our problems reside within us; it's just a matter of finding them and bringing them to the surface. Someone once approached the famous composer Sergey Rachmaninoff to ask how he came to compose his music. Rachmaninoff suggested that it was quite simple: He sat in a room by himself and listened to the music; when it stopped, he simply recorded it on paper. This bears witness to the enormous value of meditation and silent reflection as a means of recovering the wisdom of one's inner self.

The individuation journey is hard work and is strewn with potholes. It takes courage to take actions that contradict social norms. Often, self-awareness resurrects grief and terrifying feelings. Jim remembers the first time someone called his attention to his morbidlike laugh, a disturbing revelation that caused him anguish for more than a few weeks until he became conscious of similar laughter by most people, at least occasionally and especially in response to a "sick" joke. A former nurse, who is now a practice management consultant, reports that it is common to hear morbid humor

> *"[I]f we imagine this being [an individual] as a larger or smaller room, it is obvious that most people come to know only one corner of their room, one spot near the window, one narrow strip on which they keep walking back and forth."*[6]
>
> —Rainer Maria Rilke
>
>

in the emergency or operating room as a way of relieving stress.

Many people don't care to look into their soul because of religious upbringing. For years, they may have been exposed to the belief that we are really wretched creatures. Until its service book was revised in the late 1970s, one mainstream Protestant denomination included as part of the confession, "We poor sinners confess unto Thee that we are by nature sinful and unclean." Similar forms of theology can be found in almost every religious discipline and causes people to fear their shadows.

Your Golden Shadow

A word coined by Carl Jung, *shadow* is often the repressed, dark side of personality. Everyone has a shadow. It has to do with the principle of opposites. When we identify with some aspect of ourselves in our conscious personality ("I am a hard worker" or "I am honest"), the opposite is also true and often resides in the unconscious. Every perception, belief, or truth has a counterpart.

The shadow, or underground side of personality, develops at an early age. A newborn has a 360-degree personality: all aspects of the infant are exposed. Then parents begin to look at the child, making decisions about aspects of the child that are acceptable and about behavior that is not allowable. If a parent says, "You're too noisy," then the noisy part of the child goes underground into the shadow. When the child enters school, teachers and classmates make judgments about the child's personality, and additional aspects of the child are repressed into the shadow. Things that we are not supposed to be or do go underground. They can be our happiness, laziness, craziness, creativity, sexuality, and so on. More often than not, people view the shadow as dark and evil, but Jung viewed the shadow as 90 percent gold. The plodding, keep-your-nose-to-the-grindstone person, always carrying a burden, has residing within her or him a dancing, singing, lighthearted, don't-forget-to-smell-the-roses shadow. Figure 5-2 is a worksheet designed to identify your shadow elements.

FIGURE 5-2

Identifying Your Shadows Worksheet

In the space below, identify some personal beliefs/principles, then state their opposites. They may include some of the beliefs previously identified as having come from your parents. They may also include known strengths and skills. The opposites may reflect parts of your shadow.

To experience your shadow, act upon it. For example, if a parent's advice admonishes you to "work hard and keep your nose to the grindstone," some weekend do nothing that requires work. This may require courage because of the fear involved and because you are violating powerful parental messages. However, it may have a liberating impact on your life.

Personal Beliefs/Principles	Their Opposites (Shadow)
Examples:	
Be good	*Bad feelings, nasty impulses*
Always do your best	*Perfectionism—your best is never good enough—relax—take it easy*
Be successful	*Failure is a wonderful learning experience.*

Example of the Golden Shadow   From the time Sally was a young child, her parents psychologically abused her. They claimed she was clumsy and inept and would never amount to anything. Her wealthy parents even went so far as to set up a trust fund for her living expenses. Sally's anger about these messages surfaced immediately when she engaged a career counselor. The results from some career assessment instruments failed to evoke any genuine vocational enthusiasm, so her counselor decided to probe more deeply through an interview process.

Counselor: Describe a typical day in your life.
Sally: Well, I get up about 7 A.M. and have breakfast.
Counselor: Then what do you do?
Sally: I take a walk.
Counselor: OK, but what about the rest of your day? What do you do that's interesting?
Sally: Nothing much, I suppose.

This conversation continued for a lengthy period until the counselor was about to give up. Perhaps her parents were right. Sally could be totally inept.

Counselor: Come on, Sally, there must be something you enjoy.
Sally: Well, I do like to read sports magazines.

Eureka! After probing this subject more intently, it turned out that Sally was a sports trivia nut. She knew that Roger Staubach grew an inch when he was a senior in high school. Sally's golden shadow was uncovered. Residing in Texas, she was sent for a visit to the Texas Sports Hall of Fame, where she eventually landed a part-time job cataloging sports information.

Example of the Dark Shadow   One person reported how on a Monday morning word spread like wildfire across the factory floor that Ralph's office was empty. Ralph was a command and

control production manager of
a medium-sized manufacturing
facility; his attitude was hard-
ened by years of hard-nosed
production demands. He required absolute loyalty from his
employees and impeccable honesty. Ralph served as an elder in
his local church, sometimes
preaching in the absence of his
pastor. He prided himself on
being a respected leader in the
community and had served as
president of the Lion's Club.

> *"Refusing to accept
> shadow elements and
> continuing to deny their
> presence in ourselves
> makes us less than whole
> persons. Trying to appear
> to be 'better' than we are
> prevents our becoming
> what we can be."*[7]
>
> —Robert Miller
> ❧

Now he was gone and eventually the story surfaced. It seems
that Ralph made arrangements with a contractor to resurface the
roof of the manufacturing plant. As part of the deal, he instructed
the roofer to repair his home as well and hide the cost as part of the
expense of the factory job. An employee in the accounting department discovered the extra expense and reported it to the plant
manager. Ralph was terminated, a victim of his shadow and the
inability to see his whole self.

CODEPENDENCE AND DIFFERENTIATION

Codependence is an emotional state based on a reliance on
someone or something else for one's well-being. Codependent
workers allow external sources to control them while they trust
their needs will be met. Even as entitlements begin to vanish in
today's competitive market environment, they tolerate uncertainty for the sake of a steady paycheck. They become paralyzed
by organizational and vocational change. Instead of working
constructively through the grief process to renewal, codependent

workers recycle from depression to denial, anger, fear, and back to depression again.

Corbin suggests that organizational codependence exposes itself in at least five ways:[8]

1. A willingness to sacrifice one's best interests for the sake of external praise
2. Withdrawal from significant interactions with fellow employees
3. An unrealistic belief that one can solve the problems of others and rescue them
4. Refusal to acknowledge and discuss stress-related problems
5. Fearful immobilization caused by the assumption that one has a right to job security

For many years, corporations have fostered codependency through paternalism and by encouraging workers to assume life-long employment and entitlement to benefits. Paradoxically, considering the entire history of humankind, this has been the *only* period when job security has been a factor and a possibility for the masses of people. However, this momentary ride through a very temporary period in history is ending.

Self-differentiation stands in radical contrast to codependence. Self-directed people are guided by internal gyroscopes. They have a keen discernment of their personal strengths and weaknesses. Feelings across the wide spectrum of emotion are accepted as normal and necessary and are expressed when and if appropriate. Self-directed people view downturns and misfortunes caused by organizational change as temporary or even as opportunities.

A brief summary of the nature of self-differentiation as compared with codependence is shown in table 5-1.

Words such as *depth, meaning, connectedness,* and *receptivity* that describe soul also describe self-differentiation, even though this doesn't mean that codependence is the antithesis of soul. Almost everyone displays codependent behavior at times, depending on the circumstance. Soul embraces the messiness as well as the

TABLE 5-1

Characteristics of Codependence and Self-Differentiation

Codependence	Self-Differentiation
Gripped by anxiety and fear in the face of change	Intellectual system developed sufficiently to rationally respond to change
Dependent on positive feedback from others and avoids or reacts violently to negative information	Assumes responsibility, if appropriate, when positive or negative feedback is received
Particularly in management, seeks to control others or situations to minimize personal fear	Fosters problem solving when faced with difficulty, expresses empathy, and seeks to negotiate solutions to problems
Vague about long-term goals ("I just want to be happy.")	Clear vision of organizational and/or personal, vocational direction
Uses indirect tactics in an attempt to manipulate unpleasant situations	Approaches difficulty directly and assertively

cleanliness of life. It resides in the peaks and valleys, the light and the darkness of daily experience. If there is an antithesis to soul, it might be denial—an unwillingness to face and experience the complexity of life and work.

As we have said, recalling and retelling your unique, personal story enhances soul. The mind functions more like an intriguing rain forest than like a computer. Like a rain forest, endless, shadowy places are there to explore, and an energy propels us toward growth and individuation. This energy encourages us to differentiate ourselves from others. It sets the stage for exploring our career stories and for uncovering a sense of unique vocational calling.

References
[1] Thomas Moore, *Care of the Soul* (New York: HarperCollins, 1992), p. xvi.

2 Rachel Naomi Remen, *Kitchen Table Wisdom* (New York: River-head Books, 1996), p. xxv.

3 Richard Stone, *StoryWork Institute Newsletter* (winter/spring 1998): 6.

4 Tom Chappell, *The Soul of a Business* (New York: Bantam Books, 1993), p. 60.

5 June Singer, *Boundaries of the Soul* (Garden City, N.Y.: Anchor Books, 1973).

6 Rainer Maria Rilke, *Letters to a Young Poet* (New York: Vintage Books, 1984), p. 90.

7 Robert Miller, *Your Golden Shadow* (San Francisco: Harper & Row, 1989), p. 74.

8 Carolyn Corbin, *Conquering Corporate Codependence* (Engelwood Cliffs, N.J.: Prentice Hall Trade, 1993).

CHAPTER SIX

Soul and Vocation

*"Dad, I can't stand it any more. Maybe [college
is] . . . all right for some fellows. But me, I want
to get into mechanics."
"Well . . . now, for heaven's sake, don't repeat
this to your mother . . . but practically, I've
never done a single thing I've wanted to in my
whole life."*[1]

—Sinclair Lewis, *Babbitt*

*W*hen he was 12 years old, Jim's son, David, ventured on a solo
trip to Washington, D.C., to visit his uncle, who promptly swept
him away to Chesapeake Bay for a day of sailing on a 19-foot sailboat. After this experience, David was hooked on sailing for life
and was soon devouring sailing magazines and nagging his father to
take him to local marinas.

The following spring, David's parents finally succumbed to his
newly found passion and bought him a tiny Sears Styrofoam Sun-
flower. Of course, much to their consternation, David had to
launch the boat the same day it was purchased, even though winds
were gusting to 25 mph. He was okay on the downwind leg but was
unable to tack through the wind on the return trip without tum-
bling into the water.

While his parents watched, petrified with fear, eventually a motorboat driver cast him a line and hauled him to shore. Feeling like a salty old sailor on reaching shore, David leaped from his boat and exclaimed, "Well, Dad, it's hard work, but I love it!"

Sailing requires money, especially if one aspires to a larger vessel. So David got himself a job at a local amusement park walking children on horses around in a circle and cleaning up after the horses. After about six weeks, the monotony and smell of manure got to him and he finally quit. He then announced that the following year he would find satisfying employment. His parents silently chuckled, knowing from their own experience that it usually requires years of preparation and perseverance to come anywhere close to finding work that is enjoyable.

One early evening the following summer, however, David burst through the garage door into the kitchen. He had visited a downtown loft and announced he hired on as an apprentice sailmaker. Sailmaking is hard, precise work, but for David it was virtually child's play. Each morning he would gleefully leave the house, invigorated by the deep pleasure of his work as compared with the previous year's drudgery of horse tending. The former was just a job. Now, he had soul work.

SOULFUL WORK AND VOCATIONAL CALLING

The word *opus* in Latin means "to work." Also associated with music, opus suggests that soulful work has something to do with rhythm and harmony. Like the seven dwarfs, friends of Snow White, it is to "whistle while you work."

Notwithstanding that the labor may be painstaking, soulful work calls us to pursue certain tasks with passion. Many health care professionals, driven by a passion for a specialty, work many hard years to become licensed practitioners. The time and effort they expend remains tolerable because the work they pursue generates emotion, even love.

The story is told of one physician who, reflecting later on his experience as a medical student, reported his awe at the responsibility he had and his continuing amazement that he was being paid for the privilege of learning about and sharing the lives of other people.

The word *vocation* means "calling." In our estimation, one's vocational calling manifests itself in at least three dimensions. The first involves the heavy work and lifelong journey of becoming fully human. It is to know oneself, individuate, and become as humanly conscious as possible.

The second component of calling involves the serious work of being a caring, socially responsible participant in the local, national, and world community. In religious terminology, it is to love one's neighbor, including the environment. In *What Color Is Your Parachute?* it means "to do what you can, moment by moment, day by day, step by step, to make this world a better place."[2]

The third part of calling embraces the work of discovering and pursuing the soul's vocational calling in relation to one's unique gifts and talents, the focus of this chapter. In his bestseller *The Soul's Code,* Hillman suggests that just as an acorn knows instinctively what it means to become an oak tree, so, too, we have a unique, genetic instinct of what we were placed here on earth to accomplish. "There is more in a human life than our theories of it allow. Sooner or later something seems to call us onto a particular path. You may remember this 'something' as a signal moment in childhood when an urge out of nowhere, a fascination, a peculiar turn of events struck like an annunciation: This is what I must do, this is what I've got to have. This is who I am."[3]

Although not usually associating soul with a vocational calling until recently, career development professionals for years have helped people to identify and pursue a soulful career path. "The ultimate care of the soul is having work that you love," suggests Dr. Helen Harkness of Career Design Associates in Garland, Texas. "You don't have to be good at everything, just that which feeds the soul."

Dr. Fred Otte, professor of vocational and career development at Georgia State University in Atlanta, concurs. "To me, soul, spirituality, and vocation can't be separated. When people are out of touch with the deepest parts of themselves, they and their employers lose a vital resource. It's not uncommon today for people to be searching for their own spiritual path and organizing the rest of their lives around it, particularly after middle age."

> *"I think the person who takes a job in order to live—that is to say, [just] for money—has turned himself into a slave."*
>
> —Joseph Campbell
>
>

According to Moore, "Sometimes we refer to work as an 'occupation,' an engaging word meaning 'to be taken and seized.' . . . Most people can tell ill-fated stories of how they happened to end up in their current 'occupation.'"[4] Often, people also feel "seized" by their jobs in the negative sense of dreading to return to work on Monday.

A job may mean engaging in distasteful tasks for the sole purpose of paying the bills. A job conjures up images of procrastination in beginning the day. The highlight of the morning may be the coffee break; the afternoon is filled with clock watching; and the evening is devoted to overindulgence in food, drink, or TV to compensate for the stress or boredom of the day.

One physician noted that the majority of his patients suffer greatly from frustration and dissatisfaction in their jobs. Yet medical history as usually taken simply reduces a patient's work life as a line on a form marked "Occupation"—just one more way in which our stories are not encouraged (as discussed in chapter 5).

Job Versus Vocation

All of us have jobs to do. Someone must bring home the bread, carry out the garbage, and mow the lawn, but if we perform soul-diminishing tasks for days and weeks, we are headed for physical and emotional trouble.

Some time ago, Jim's boss handed him a new and, unfortunately, soulless temporary assignment. The company needed approval for a rate increase from the Public Utility Commission; for the commission hearings, 27 one-inch to three-inch binders of material were prepared with 100 copies of each binder. Jim's boss volunteered his services to help in proofing the binders to ensure that no material was misplaced. Though fairly competent at it, Jim hates to proofread, especially material that is about as dull and dry as a desert acre.

> "*Work is love made visible.*"
>
> —Khalil Gibran
>
> ✒

He made it through the first day of the assignment but called in sick the second day (in retrospect, it was vocational soul sickness). During the morning of the third day, Jim received an out-of-the-blue, urgent phone call requesting vocational counseling and outplacement services because of a major plant layoff. Thereafter, Jim became so busy performing his permanent job that he was unable to return to the soulless job of proofing binders.

On the other hand, work as vocation is something we are drawn into because it excites us and is fulfilling. For many people, raising children, woodworking, gardening, leading Boy Scouts or Girl Scouts, or simply listening to a friend serves as soulful work. It is often work we love to do when we have leisure time on our hands.

We can see that vocation has a broader dimension; it's not just your job or your occupation, although it may include both. Rather, it is something that shapes your leisure, your relationships, your private life, and your public life. It is something that orchestrates much of your waking time.

The Distinguishing Characteristics of Soulful Work
Work versus a job—how can we distinguish one from the other?
What follows are questions that indicate criteria to help you differ-
entiate between the two:

- *What are you doing when time seems to fly?* When engaged in
  soulful work activities, either on or off the job, time seems to pass
  quickly. An hour seems like 10 minutes because we are so
  intently engaged.
- *What activity captivates your childlike playful passion?* In other
  words, you undoubtedly pursue this activity whether or not you
  are earning money. Turning this venture into a moneymaking
  enterprise could become a career goal.
- *What type of work summons your energy and enthusiasm?* Enthusiasm taps the rich resources of the soul. It is a word that literally
  means to be "in God."
- *What undertaking becomes the focus of your creative impulse?*
  Engaging in creative work is another way to nourish the soul.
  Creativity is an instinct common to everyone. It can manifest
  itself not only in art but in everything we do, including work and
  leisure.
- *What essential gift(s) do you wish to give to the world?* Most of us
  want to feel that what we do in terms of work makes a significant
  difference. We would like to leave a legacy when we die.

HOW TO IDENTIFY YOUR CAREER MISSION

*T*he concepts of vocational calling and career mission are virtually
interchangeable. The concept of career mission leans a bit more on
the side of one's specific occupation or job. It describes the basic
arena of one's daily work. Just as a corporation must clearly
describe the basic nature of its business, it is helpful for individuals
to describe their personal career mission.

Over the years, Jim refined his career assessment process, as shown in figure 6-1. Career assessment can be a lengthy process that sometimes involves months of work. Because many people are constrained by time, money, or limited motivation to engage in a lengthy evaluation process, Jim commonly uses four basic assessment instruments. The first is a functional skills inventory, identifying key, transferable, satisfying skills used frequently on or off the job. Ten or so key skills are listed in the order of their priority to identify skills which are so vital to each client that they must be used both on and off the job. In Jim's experience, people become very stressed, sometimes even physically sick, if they are unable to apply these skills in daily work.

The second instrument is the Myers-Briggs Type Indicator (MBTI®). Two American women, Katharine Briggs and her gifted daughter, Isabel Briggs Myers, gathered information that evolved

FIGURE 6-1

Career Development Model

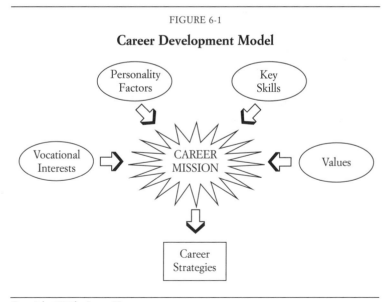

into the MBTI®, which today represents the most widely used instrument of its kind in the world to focus primarily on personality preferences and strengths. You may even be able to complete the assessment instrument on the Internet, possibly at no cost (keyword: Myers-Briggs). After identifying a client's profile using the MBTI®, Jim refers to the book *Do What You Are,* which relates each of 16 possible personality types to careers.[5] Jim considers this excellent book one of the key career assessment resources available.

Third, clients complete *The Self-Directed Search* or some other version of John Holland's six types of careers.[6] Career consultant pioneers John Holland and Richard Bolles popularized the idea of individuals attending an imaginary vocational party where they converse and discuss six types of careers based on common vocational interests. The six career areas are:

- *Artistic:* people who are especially creative in artistic endeavors. They could be actors, painters, sculptors, writers, or computer graphic designers.
- *Social:* those who like to interface with others and provide some kind of service. Occupations may include sales, customer service, teaching, counseling, or many human resource fields in business.
- *Investigative:* people who like to learn, observe, analyze situations and data, and solve problems. They could be scientists, police investigators, physicians, systems analysts, or technicians.
- *Realistic:* those who are more often outdoor types—"hands-on" individuals who enjoy working with objects, tools, plants, or animals. They could be farmers, mechanics, construction workers, plumbers, or hardware store clerks and managers.
- *Conventional:* people who generally enjoy routine, steady kinds of jobs and often enjoy structure and detail work. They could be secretaries, accountants, data entry specialists, or assembly workers.
- *Enterprising:* people who enjoy discussing their entrepreneurial interests and who might be in business for themselves or work as managers, stockbrokers, or explorers.

The fourth exercise assists in identifying significant work values and uses *Career Anchors,* designed by Edgar H. Schein of the Massachusetts Institute of Technology (MIT).[7] Think of a boat anchored to the bottom of a lake that shifts around in a circle according to the direction of the wind but remains essentially in one place, although the boat drifts away if the anchor line is severed. Schein identifies eight career anchors:

1. Technical/functional competence
2. Managerial competence
3. Autonomy/independence
4. Security/stability
5. Entrepreneurship/creativity
6. Service/dedication
7. Pure challenge
8. Lifestyle integration

Schein's instrument allows you to identify your most important anchors. If, like the boat, your career anchor is severed because of a change in the work environment, you may lose your way. Many medical professionals, as noted earlier, value autonomy and independence, values being undermined by the changing tide of health care. Also, a desire to provide a medical service can be significantly diminished by management pressures to limit visits to 6 to 10 minutes.

The feedback from the four career assessment instruments generally allows the individual being assessed to construct a statement of career mission. From this sense of mission, specific career strategies can be formulated and implemented.

The Importance of Career Mission

Having a personal sense of career mission can contribute to one's overall physical and mental health. In *The Will to Live,* Hutschnecker reminds us of Goethe's belief that every extraordinary man has a mission he is called upon to fulfill.[8] The same

Sir Thomas More: *But Richard . . . Why not be a teacher? You'd be a fine teacher. Perhaps even a great one.* Richard: *And if I was, who would know it?* Sir Thomas: *You, your pupils, your friends, God. Not a bad public. . . .*

—Robert Bolt

holds true for ordinary men and women. Considering that each one of us lives for such a short period, having meaning and purpose in life along with a sense of making a difference undoubtedly contributes to both the quality and length of one's life.

Hans Selye, generally regarded as the father of modern stress management, agrees: "Life must be allowed to run its natural course toward the fulfillment of its innate potential. In this sense, and to my mind, the aim of life is to maintain its own identity and express its innate abilities and drives with the least possible frustration."[9] Selye suggests that uncovering and pursuing one's life/career mission contribute to a life without significant distress and to health in general.

Your Career Journey
Many books and resources are available to help identify your vocational passion. Perhaps most widely known is Bolles' *What Color Is Your Parachute?*[10] which is revised annually. The appendix provides a sample of career counselors and other resources throughout the country. If you are motivated to find direction on your own, some things you can do include the following:

• First, identify messages regarding work and career given to you from parents and other significant adults, especially during early childhood years. These could be messages residing in your shadow, as described in chapter 5. A significant number of people end up visiting career guidance professionals because of early advice they've been given without considering their skills and aptitude. Parental figures may say, "Don't be an artist. You'll never make any money. Why don't you get into medicine or law?" So you may end up investing time and money pursuing a career inconsistent with your true calling. On the other hand, some caring adults observe children pursuing certain interests and the adults provide appropriate tutelage. In any case, it is helpful to reflect on early messages to determine if they were helpful or harmful.

For example, during his early childhood Charles published and marketed a neighborhood newspaper. Later, while in the service, he wrote for *Stars and Stripes*. Though his real love was journalism, on graduation from college, he went to work in his father's insurance agency. When his father died, Charles sold the agency and went to work for a major midwestern newspaper, where he rose through the ranks to become managing editor.

- Imagine that your soul is a wise inner self. In almost all cultures, interesting names and images are used to describe this inner wisdom. The Sioux Indians speak of the "familiar voice." Northwest Native Americans named the inner self after an animal, the wolf. (See Tara Bruin's story and poem in the appendix.) Jung himself engaged in dialogue with Philemon, his "one million-year-old man." In the Christian tradition, St. Paul used the language of the "Christ" self more than 100 times in his epistles. Zen Buddhists call it the "original face." Practice *active receptivity;* that is, ask for vocational guidance, then during the days and weeks ahead be receptive and welcome new information regarding vocational direction.

- Look through the rearview mirror of your job experiences and personal life to identify key events that were particularly satisfying. These could be accomplishments from any period of your life that were soulful in the sense that you felt deep pleasure and an energized connection to them. Try to identify at least five such accomplishments and write a paragraph describing each. Look for common themes and skills you used. You may wish to ask close friends or family members to help with this exercise.

Susan, who was quite unhappy as a medical technician, discovered that she had a history of writing with clarity and humor. She made a transfer to the hospital's communications department as an administrative assistant. Shortly after, she requested and received some writing assignments and eventually became a public relations specialist.

- Here is an activity you may remember from your earlier days. Flip through a variety of magazines, identifying and cutting out pictures that seem appealing and soulful to you. Paste them on a large piece of cardboard to make a collage. Look for patterns and themes. Again, friends could help you with this exercise as long as they aren't judgmental.

Frank, who had lost his job as a technician in a manufacturing facility, found himself drawn to people and things of beauty while constructing his collage. He eventually found a job in sales (actually more customer service) for a Lincoln Continental dealership.

- Stand behind yourself, so to speak, and observe yourself as you walk into a large bookstore. Which section first comes to your attention? Where do you go next? Could subjects of interest lead you in the direction of a vocational pursuit?

Dorothy became quite weary of the long hours associated with her job as an internist, but she had always been interested in philosophy and ethics. She decided to return to school for additional education to become a medical ethicist.

- Your organization may not offer a career development function like the one described below. However, most universities and community colleges offer career guidance for a nominal fee. This may be an excellent first step in your journey to uncover your soul's calling and career mission.

CAREER DEVELOPMENT IN HEALTH CARE

*O*ne physician's journey toward career renewal began in 1994. Todd Pearson, MD, decided to take a three-month sabbatical from a very successful pediatric practice. "The purpose of the sabbatical was expressly to address my personal sense of burnout and my growing questions and concerns regarding career 'fit,' questions that had been lurking in the recesses of my mind like a haunting refrain. . . . To use a well-worn but useful metaphor, I had climbed the ladder of success, with all its trappings, only to find it leaning against the wrong wall."[11] Also, since the beginning of his clinical education, Todd never felt at ease in what he calls the "John Wayne School of Medicine," which implies that "real" doctors should not allow themselves to be seen as vulnerable. This paradigm teaches physicians directly or indirectly to be tough, unemotional, and private and to solve problems by overworking.

During the sabbatical, Todd immersed himself in books on diverse topics, including self-help, spirituality, career development, and leadership. He invested in himself completely, something he had never done before, at least not with the same intensity.

In addition to exploring his vocational "why," Todd began to give more quality time to his children. During the early 1990s, Todd's wife retired from nursing to be a stay-at-home mom. She thoroughly enjoyed raising the children and Todd's desire was to share more deeply in the joy of being emotionally as well as physically present for them.

During his sabbatical, he became curious about what resources might be available for health care professionals like himself. He knew that he was not the only person suffering in silence. In the Northwest, there were some career counselors whose practice included physicians, but they weren't in touch with the issues and concerns of the medical profession. Todd expanded his search nationally and began to network, seeking resources specifically for physicians. His search became an all-consuming passion, the answer to his personal "why," and became much more of a calling for him than medicine had been. During this period, he developed a vision of a center where physicians could come for renewal, a place that would address multiple human resource concerns.

Within a few months of concluding his sabbatical, Todd reduced his working hours to three-fourths of the usual time he practiced. Over the next year and a half he continued to disengage from the practice. He enrolled in a postgraduate program at the University of Washington and became certified in career development. He also received certification as a Senior Coach in Individual and Organizational Coaching with the Hudson Institute of Santa Barbara.

In 1996 Todd opened the Center for Physician Renewal in Bellevue, Washington. The center is devoted to the facilitation of life/career resilience for health care professionals and to the creation of "resilient" health care organizations. It provides insight and support for individuals experiencing career dissatisfaction, stress, burnout, and job loss. It broadens one's sense of "Who am I?" and "Who do I want to become?" The center assists individuals in defining clinical and nonclinical career options as well as illuminating and evaluating career options outside of medicine. It guides health care professionals through the climate of accelerating change, teaching them how to expand their options and avoid getting trapped in old ways of thinking. It helps people learn from the past, keeping what remains functional and satisfying in order to serve others. Finally, it offers coaching and career development resources to promote organizational effectiveness. This includes formulating and implementing strategies to create a resilient physician workforce.

Career Development at Swedish Medical Center

Founded in 1910, Swedish Medical Center, with two campuses, serves as one of the Northwest's largest and most comprehensive medical centers. In 1997 the medical center in Seattle initiated a forward-thinking program to enhance soul in the careers of its employees. As part of an expanded commitment to staff development, the center established an Employee Advancement Center, whose goal is to keep people invested and advancing in their careers, whether at Swedish or beyond, whether in health care or in another field. The assumption is that employees who are helped to identify career/life goals will be more productive in their current job. There is an adage stating, "Freedom is expanding your options." Employees who know they have choices and options are apt to work more fervently in their current jobs.

The center's director, Robert Hamilton, was quoted in the *Seattle Post-Intelligencer:* "People get very siloed in health care. People get stuck thinking 'this is all I can do.' We help people look outside the box and identify transferable skills." [12]

Some, and perhaps many, administrators and managers fear that offering career development increases the risk of losing valued workers. In most instances, however, just the opposite is true, at least in terms of workers leaving the overall organization. Most employees find themselves working in careers appropriate for their skills and interests. The career assessment process usually affirms current vocational direction, simply bringing to greater clarity key skills and strengths. In addition, people normally don't change jobs and careers unless they are experiencing acute emotional pain; for most people, the process of changing involves considerable risk and uncertainty. Therefore, career assessment usually enhances the use of key skills and knowledge in an employee's current position.

The center, available to Swedish Medical Center's 4,000 employees, offers assessment, goal setting, résumé writing, and interview preparation, all of which can be used for internal and/or external career advancement. The center's library offers titles on career planning, transitioning, communications, and the job search. An educational resource room offers curriculum catalogs from local education and training institutions. Computer workstations serve as a means to sharpen computer skills in Microsoft Word, Excel, Access, and power typing, and employees also have access to the Internet.

We are not suggesting that Swedish is or is not highly regarded for having soul. That is for others to decide. Within any organization, however, there may be such soul-enhancing programs or activities as career development.

CONCLUSION

$\mathcal{B}$ecause most people spend one-half or more of their time earning a living, addressing the issues of soul in work is vital. As French philosopher Albert Camus has written, "Without work all life goes rotten. But when work is soulless, life stifles and dies." On the other hand, soulful work arouses enthusiasm and passion in us. Like a hearty breakfast, soulful work energizes and prepares us to enjoy the day ahead.

Even if you have family and financial obligations or educational limitations that prevent you from seeking soulful work, you can prepare now for the future by pursuing your interests as an avocation. Most of us overcome obstacles and climb mountains in the same manner—one step at a time.

References

[1] Sinclair Lewis, *Babbitt* (San Diego: Harcourt Brace Jovanovich, 1922), p. 472.

[2] Richard Nelson Bolles, *What Color Is Your Parachute?* (Berkeley, Calif.: Ten Speed Press, 1998), p. 225.

[3] James Hillman, *The Soul's Code* (New York: Random House, 1996), p. 3.

[4] Thomas Moore, *Care of the Soul* (New York: HarperCollins, 1992), p. 182.

5 Paul D. Tieger and Barbara Barron-Tieger, *Do What You Are* (Boston: Little, Brown, 1995).

6 John L. Holland, *The Self-Directed Search* (Odessa, Fla.: Psychological Assessment Resources, 1990).

7 Edgar H. Schein, *Career Anchors* (San Diego: University Associates, 1990, published by Pfeiffer & Co.).

8 Arnold A. Hutschnecker, *The Will to Live* (New York: Cornerstone Library, 1978).

9 Hans Selye, *Stress without Distress* (New York: New American Library, 1974), p. 102.

10 Bolles, *Your Parachute.*

11 Richard L. Haid and Todd Pearson, "The Changing Landscape of Career Development in Medicine," *Career Planning and Adult Development Journal* (spring 1998): 7.

12 Carol Smith, "Swedish Helps Its Employees Advance toward Dream Jobs," *Seattle Post-Intelligencer* (May 15, 1998): B1.

CHAPTER SEVEN

Soul and Diversity

"We shall not cease from exploration
And the end of all our exploring
Will be to arrive where we started
And know the place for the first time." [1]

—T. S. Eliot, *Four Quartets*

$\mathcal{T}$he root of the word *cosmos* means adornment, reflecting the beauty, splendor, and awesomeness of the universe. The soul of the universe embellishes itself with wonder and diversity.

OUTER DIVERSITY

$\mathcal{O}$ur galaxy alone spins an immense pinwheel of billions of stars. Back in the late 1930s, efforts to catalog the stars of our Milky Way resulted in an estimate of 40 million. Today, astronomers have stopped counting.

Beyond our relatively small galaxy, it is estimated that more then 100 million constellations join up as our neighbors. And as if this were not enough to boggle the mind, some scientists currently speculate there may be as many as eight dimensions to the universe, not three. So we live in a multiverse, not a universe.

Closer to home, our planet thrives on an extremely thin layer of earth known as the biosphere, which includes the atmosphere. According to Pulitzer Prize winner Edward Wilson, "The most wonderful mystery of life may well be the means by which it created so much diversity from so little physical matter. The biosphere makes up only about one part in ten billion of the earth's mass."[2]

Biodiversity is the key to maintenance of the world as we know it. It refers to the wide range of different types of organisms in a given place at a given time. More than one million living animal species have currently been identified, the overwhelming number of which are insects. Species come and go at an astonishing rate. Depending on who is doing the estimating, any number of species become extinct every hour, either because of natural processes or because of human pollution and the deteriorating environment.

The health care professions prosper on nature's diversity; their disciplines are relentless explorers of body and mind. Endlessly, the diversity of life has been broken apart, described, measured, pictured, cataloged, and reassembled by physicians and scientists. For example, *Dorland's Illustrated Medical Dictionary* contains more than 1,860 pages of medical vocabulary, beginning with *Aarane,* a trademark for a preparation of cromolyn sodium, and ending with *Zymosterol,* a mycosterol occurring in yeast.

Soul flourishes on the diversity of life. It embraces the vernacular, connecting with a particular species, element, or place with all of its complexity. It inspires awe and gives birth to curiosity. It embraces that which is different, weird, spooky, quaint, unusual, and eccentric.

Diversity of Places
Have you ever visited an unusual and quaint place, perhaps a locality or region where you have never been before? Some years ago we took an autumn trip to Connecticut for the first time to visit Jim's daughter. We spent an entire day traveling through the old,

quaint towns and countryside, soaking in the October foliage and pumpkin-laden harvest atmosphere. Soul revealed herself in the weathered stone walls, the misty mornings, and the steepled churches.

Shortly after our move to the Seattle area, where we now live, we were informed that Seattle was the most unchurched city in the United States with less than 10 percent of the population attending Sunday worship. Later, someone else suggested that this region is one of the more spiritual places on earth. If so, we suspect this has something to do with the diversity of its people, places, and physical environment.

An antiseptic office, clinic, or hospital diminishes diversity and the enhancement of soul in health care. We don't mean these places must be unclean, but they can be constructed and adorned in a manner to help us feel more at home. As one medical school professor put it, buildings are usually designed by architects according to business function and the wishes of their clients. In the past, hospitals have typically not been designed in ways that enhance the comfort, needs, and care of patients.

A large 555-bed regional medical center in northern Texas grew in stages over a period of some 15 years. It includes the main hospital building and two connecting medical office buildings. In a move virtually unheard of at the time, the hospital's builder and owner (not the hospital) intentionally designed and created an environment that would not look or feel like the typical sterile, utilitarian facility. A forerunner of the medical mall concept, the lobby reminds one of a mall or hotel, with play areas for children, fountains, various food sections, and gift shops. This comfortable lobby environment has been subsequently duplicated in a smaller fashion in some of the newer office building additions. Ambulatory patients, expectant mothers awaiting delivery, and other visitors feel welcome to walk and shop. Such an atmosphere helps both patients and visitors to feel more comfortable and less fearful.

A medium-sized hospital in the Northwest has also grown over time. Looking more like a pleasant hotel, its lobby affords an atmosphere of serenity and peace. Colors are softly muted and a glass-enclosed plant area is central to the main lobby. The hospital throughout suggests calmness and caring.

Diversity of People

To be truly human and mature involves embracing the opposites in life. The universe thrives on polarity. We have two eyes, ears, hands, and so on. Polarity allows us to set aside someone or something for the purposes of contrast and definition. We would not know what it means to be a woman if it were not for men. Right is contrary to wrong, health to disease, joy to sorrow, profit to loss. Soul too prospers on differences.

Just as learning to speak different languages enriches one's vocabulary and understanding of the meaning of words, establishing relationships with diverse groups of people enhances the experience of soul. Because most health care organizations provide services to a dissimilar customer/client base, diversity is especially important in the health care workplace. A diverse workplace welcomes African Americans, Native Americans, Asian Americans, Latinos, recent immigrants, Jews, Muslims, the disabled, younger and older workers, men and women, gays and lesbians.

In *The Soul of a Business,* Chappell states, "We have learned to see that hiring and having differences within the company—not just the color of people's skin or in their accent, but in their education, their experience, their background, and their abilities—is a business advantage, a major business advantage, besides being a moral responsibility."[3]

Diversity in Organizations

Diversity leads to organizational effectiveness in the following ways:

- It brings a richness of perspective and creativity to the organization. Health care in particular and business in general are becoming increasingly complex. A diversity of eyes and ears widens our view of any given issue or opportunity.
- It provides a heightened sensitivity to the diversity of an organization's customer base. Can you imagine how uncomfortable it could be for a minority person to enter a strange hospital whose staff was made up of only white men or women of approximately the same age?
- It leads to a more complete utilization of expensive human resources. By the year 2000, 85 percent of the entering workforce will be female, African American, Asian American, Latino, or new immigrants. Diversity broadens the scope of recruiting efforts and is especially important during periods of low unemployment.
- It increases the awareness and need for effective communication skills and techniques. Sensitivity to cultural differences increases with variety.
- It sensitizes the organization to its legal, moral, and social responsibility. The sight of a diverse workgroup can actually minimize a client's fear of being discriminated against.

INNER DIVERSITY

*W*hat it means to be an individual includes the vast unknown (see chapter 5). Much of who we are remains concealed to us, but an individuation process is at work in the psyche, an energy challenging us to explore the unconscious and bring its vast treasures to light.

The individuation process is like a pond that is initially muddy for one reason or another. As time passes, the water becomes clearer and translucent, so you can see through it from one part to another. In human terms, individuation is the process of evolving from unconsciousness to discernment and self-realization.

Carl Jung coined the word *archetype* to describe some of the elements from unknown sources that erupt upon us from time to time. Archetypes are not static principles but life energies and images embedded in our genes. They represent primordial figures existing in the psyche down through the centuries.

An example from the animal world would be the finches on the Galapagos Islands in the Pacific Ocean. There had been no hawks on these islands for thousands of years, but when some of the finches were brought to California, they flew for cover when they saw the shadow of a hawk. The image of the hawk had been carried in the genes.

In a similar manner, we come into the world already programmed to experience things in certain ways. A newborn baby, for example, instinctively knows how to react to its mother. The archetype of mother is embedded within the child. There are a great number of such images: father, daughter, son, shadow, hero, crone (wise woman), witch, shaman (healer), wise man. Animal figures emerge as archetypes as well, such as the snake winding its way around a sword to form the medical symbol of the caduceus.

Archetypes significantly influence our assumptions, plans, and aspirations. Understood and managed in a business and/or health care environment, their power contributes to soul, productivity, creativity, and the competitive edge. When denied or suppressed, like a fierce storm they often unleash their power in very destructive ways. Some archetypes carry sufficient power to bankrupt entire organizations when misunderstood and unappreciated.

This power applies especially to the archetypes of masculine and feminine that represent fundamental images high up on the hierarchy in terms of their energy and influence. When understood and integrated in an individual or organization, the archetypes of masculine and feminine generate immense strength leading to great achievements. On the other hand, when ignored or discounted, they spawn fright and often flight.

We don't refer here to biological aspects of maleness or femaleness but to energies residing in every human. In Eastern thought, the energies are described as Yang (masculine) and Yin (feminine). Every woman bears within her the full complement of masculine energy. The reverse holds true for every man, although masculine qualities tend to be more visible and dominant because we've lived in a patriarchal culture for many centuries.

We are making the case that profitability, and perhaps even sheer survival, depend on a deepening appreciation of the feminine and the authentic marriage of the two energies. The common command and control powers of the masculine cannot function alone in an age of complex systems and the proliferation of information. An example of the extreme perversion of the masculine is ruthless and cruel behavior in business by a CEO that brings about short-term gain but long-term diminishing returns on investment (some of you may have read about "Chainsaw Al").

MASCULINE AND FEMININE ENERGIES

*M*asculine and feminine qualities as five sets of opposites are shown in figure 7-1, with masculine qualities on the left and feminine qualities on the right. They represent only a few of many descriptors, but are chosen here because of their application to health care and business in general.

We begin with the undifferentiated, unconscious unity of Yang and Yin. Feminine and masculine archetypes reside in both women and men, just as our parents gave birth to us through the creative union of egg and sperm. The sperm actively engaged the receptive egg, forming a new creation. These active and receptive characteristics, along with others, remain within us throughout life, but masculine characteristics generally go underground during the initial socialization process of women just as feminine characteristics recede into a male's unconscious. Nonetheless, these energies remain

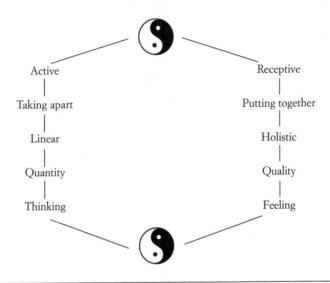

FIGURE 7-1

Qualities of Masculine/Feminine

Active	Receptive
Taking apart	Putting together
Linear	Holistic
Quantity	Quality
Thinking	Feeling

just as powerful in this underground state, whether we are aware of them or not.

Like the sperm, the masculine is active. The orientation focuses on the completion of tasks and the achievement of end results. Masculine energy in health care professionals seeks to promote well-being and healing. It includes the relentless investigation of disease and management's desire to improve productivity and gain market share.

If overextended, however, masculine energy may emerge as an overuse of status and power. When a crisis appears, the male (or female) health care professional may "damn the torpedoes, full steam ahead," and within complex medical and business systems, the torpedoes often win. Later, some of these torpedoes may explode, creating the next crisis as quickly made mergers or alliances unravel.

Such energy overextended may also apply to changing hospital boards. Most hospitals have a board of trustees whose understanding and support are critical to the organization's endeavors. Occasionally, however, one board approves the hospital's direction while incoming members are unaware of previous planning. Even with some carryover, seasoned members may not be sufficiently able to articulate the rationale behind previous decisions. Faced with new problems, well-meaning members may jump to quick, short-term fixes rather than stepping back to look at the overall picture.

One hospital faced this problem. The former board had spent considerable time and money developing a five-year strategic plan, but before the longer-term objectives could be fully implemented, the board structure changed. Carryover members weren't able to convey the story of how they had arrived at their decisions. What had been a cooperative, supportive atmosphere quickly deteriorated into an adversarial relationship between the board and the previously successful administration. Fortunately, the hospital administration understood the dynamics involved and began ongoing board development.

The opposite of the active masculine energy is the receptive feminine. Like the egg, it represents an openness and responsiveness to impending events and information, standing ready and willing to receive and nurture that which is given.

Obviously, receptivity is a key skill vital to effective intervention. To practice effectively, the health care professional must be receptive to the information and complaints of the

> *"Sometimes the greatest acts of commitment involve doing nothing but sitting and waiting until I know what to do next."*
>
> —Peter Senge
>
>

patient. In terms of management, receptivity takes the form of managing by getting around, asking questions, and listening. It spawns an open-door policy and finds expression in employee and customer opinion surveys.

But again, if overextended, receptivity can lead to a kind of passivity, becoming excessively accommodating, especially in the face of conflict. Or too much time and energy are spent on process, as opposed to content and decisiveness. Often in the presence of steamrolling, command and control managers, employees become doormats, hiding their feelings and withholding information for fear of being flattened.

Another characteristic of masculine energy is the dynamic of taking apart. In a micro sense, the health care professional is continuously taking apart, dissecting nature and the human body, examining individual components of a system. Taking something apart serves us well in problem solving and getting past vague generalizations, such as "We've got a morale problem." On the other hand, taking apart, if overextended, could lead to nitpicking, becoming overly concerned with particulars. It leads to the inability to tell the forest from the trees.

Putting together operates as a feminine alternative, having to do with understanding the interconnectedness of people, data, and objects. For the surgeon, it means putting back together that which was taken apart. For a medical technician, it involves understanding the interrelationship of biological systems with other structures. In terms of management, it encompasses a participatory style of operating, emphasizing team building and seeking consensus.

If putting together is overextended, energy is expended in the attempt to please everyone or gain the entire group's acceptance of a course of action. Managers overly concerned with being liked may sacrifice their individuality, lacking the courage to stand firm in the midst of opposition and taking the road less traveled.

Next, masculine power tends to operate in a linear fashion. It utilizes step-by-step sequential thinking, such as that involved in a serial operating procedure. Concern focuses, for example, on the length of time required to complete a task. Linear thinking tends to be one-dimensional, and if overextended, linear energy can lead to tunnel vision and inflexibility. It might cause a person to become so focused on the task at hand that he (or she) ignores the "why" questions ("Why am I doing this in the first place?").

The opposite of linear thinking is a holistic, multidimensional approach to work and business. It is seeing the whole as greater than the sum of its parts. In one sense, reclaiming soul in health care demands embracing a holistic viewpoint. It emphasizes systems thinking, seeing the impact of one part or decision on the entire enterprise. At the individual level, it involves understanding and acting on the premise that one always does make a difference, however small, in the overall scheme of things. Holistic vision, if overextended, could become a kind of passion impervious to the practicalities of the day—the inability to pay attention to detail or to understand the time and effort required to get somewhere.

The next two sets of opposites surface as a hotbed of controversy in health care. Quantity refers to concern for the amount, bulk, or body of something; today, for example, many physicians share a deep concern about assembly-line, time-pressured health care. Without an appropriate centering of attention on quantity and production, output and outcomes, and quotas and profit, however, many organizations will simply cease to exist. Almost everyone understands the problem of quantity overextended: an obsession with short-term results that devastates the caring dimension of health care.

Quality displays a rich interest in excellence and worth that's reflected in the slogan, "If it's worth doing, it's worth doing right." Obviously, few people would be attracted to a health care practitioner or institution known for inferior service. If overextended, the quality of performance could turn into nitpicking perfectionism. Contrary to the slogan, not everything worth doing is worth doing right. Time restraints in particular affect the quality of work. For example, during a medical emergency involving large numbers of people, hospital personnel do the best they can in the emergency room. Priorities must be established.

Finally, masculine energy reflects the quality of thinking. It uses logical analysis, the intellect, and critical judgment. The thinking function dominates business, especially in activities unrelated to customer or patient service. If thinking is overextended, it might cause an individual to come across as cold and impersonal. Especially during crises, many insensitivities exhibited toward people stem from management's use of icy reasoning.

Feeling obviously involves the expression of emotion and sentiment, but feeling resonates with broader qualities. It also has to do with making decisions based on their impact on others. A feeling orientation values people and acts in their best interest. Feeling, if overextended, becomes excessive caretaking. Its emphasis on being one happy family or work group could easily cause problems to be swept under the rug.

Hard-nosed, bottom-line, commonsense, thinking types in health care and business may reject the above descriptions as too subjective, theoretical, and a waste of time. Such judgments mirror the current, overwhelmingly masculine nature of many organizations, but undervaluing the feminine is like cutting off one leg. As demonstrated above, masculine characteristics unbalanced by the feminine often result in overly aggressive, controlling, and manipulative behavior. By most enlightened management standards, nitpicking, tunnel vision, and obsession with short-term results leads to deteriorating customer relations and profitability over the long haul.

Paradoxically, undervaluing and repressing the feminine side actually increases its power. Its energy goes beyond control. Like a volcano, for example, incidents of sexual harassment generally erupt from a repressed, feminine component, which is even true when the harassment was unintentional. Statements such as "I didn't know I said anything offensive" reveal an insensitivity to a part of oneself as well as to another person. Because 80 percent of health care workers are women, and the number of female medical school enrollees is now more than 40 percent, discernment of feminine energy becomes even more vital.

On the other hand, soft-hearted, accommodating, and overly friendly people may be significantly controlled by the feminine element. Their need for community and relationships overpowers their ability to attain significant results. Because the masculine element remains unclaimed and its power unavailable, such a person, who could be either a man or woman, becomes passive and submissive.

Feminine and masculine *working together* give an organization a powerful competitive edge (see figure 7-2). This synergistic, cooperative approach offers health care the flexibility to respond according to the requirements of the situation. The workings of the human eye provide an excellent example. We can see because

---

FIGURE 7-2

Masculine and Feminine Working Together

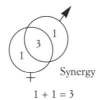

Synergy

$1 + 1 = 3$

of the focused, linear ability of the eye and because of peripheral vision. Through the eye we see both content and context. So it is with masculine and feminine components. In work situations, they allow us to concentrate on appropriate decisions. In addition, we can understand and appreciate the impact of these decisions on clients and customers, the larger workforce, and business systems.

Returning to figure 7-1, at the bottom we view again the integrated symbol for Yang and Yin. However, having been made aware of their respective qualities through this educational process and through experience, we have greater access to all of them. One's range of choices is expanded. Table 7-1 briefly describes when it is appropriate to use these masculine and feminine energies in organizations.

TABLE 7-1

When to Enlist Masculine and Feminine Energies

Masculine Skills	Feminine Skills
When time is short and action is required	When one has little or no influence or control over others
When change requires detailed analysis	When change significantly affects others
When the cause of a problem is clear	When the cause of a problem cannot be determined (Let it incubate!)
When alternatives are clear-cut	When alternatives need to be expanded
When there is not enough structure to a project or task	When there is too much structure to a project or task
When speed and timeliness are of the essence	When quality and customer satisfaction are of the essence
When brute strength is required	When long-term endurance is required

---

SOUL, DIVERSITY, AND CREATIVITY

*S*oul often expresses itself through creativity, and most of us yearn to be creative. Creativity springs from the linking and balancing of the feminine and the masculine. Again, it rises from active receptivity.

Creativity obviously derives from the word *creation* and means to make something new, so it is an active process. However, new ideas and information almost always emerge from a receptivity to the previously unknown. Creative people instinctively know and accept the reality that we don't know where we are going all of the time. Thus we act but at the same time are receptive.

An excellent, concrete example of active receptivity is the question. To actively question is to seek information, ideas, and opinions from others. Unless we are attempting to trick others by asking when we already know the answer, questioning naturally engages our receptivity.

According to Ray and Myers, "Implicitly or explicitly, creativity always begins with a question. And in both your business and personal lives, the quality of your creativity is determined by the quality of your questions—by the way you frame your approach to circumstances, needs and opportunities."[4]

Unless we are seeking concrete and factual data, open-ended questions, like open-ended stories, serve best to generate creativity. They open us to an exploration of the depth and expanse of the universe.

Two examples of the transformational integration of feminine/masculine energies follow; the first is fictional and the second is a real-life story.

Tootsie

Granted, it's a movie and a comedy at that, but in its own hilarious way, *Tootsie* demonstrates the moving of masculine and feminine energy. Michael Dorsey (played by Dustin Hoffman) patrols the booking agencies looking for an acting job. Unfortunately, his reputation as a rather brash and opinionated performer shadows him from one unsuccessful contact to another. No one will hire him because he challenges the interpretations that directors give to the characters in movies, plays, and TV dramas.

> *"[T]ry to love* the questions themselves *as if they were locked rooms or books written in a very foreign language. Don't search for the answers, which could not be given to you now, because you would not be able to live them. And the point is, to live everything. Live the questions now. Perhaps then, someday far in the future, you will gradually, without even noticing it, live your way into the answer."*[5]
>
> —Rainer Maria Rilke
>
>

When Michael learns about a casting for a soap opera about the hypothetical Southwest General Hospital, he dresses up and cosmetically transforms himself into a woman named Dorothy in order to overcome people's perceptions of him and auditions for the role of the hospital administrator.

At first, the director of the soap opera rejects Dorothy for the part, seeing her as "too soft and gentle." He's looking for a woman who acts more like a man, more appropriate for the tough job of administrator, but Dorothy is no doormat. "So you want to see some gross characteristics of a woman to prove that power makes women masculine?" At which point Dorothy abruptly lifts her knee between the director's legs and into his groin.

Dorothy not only gets the part but begins to integrate her masculine and feminine energies as she interprets the role of the hospital administrator. She is both thinking and feeling, assertive and gentle according to the situation at hand. Her performance catches the attention of the audience, especially the women, and the soap opera's ratings catapult to the top.

Dorothy's nemesis at the hospital is Dr. Brewster, who appears enamored with himself and his position. He treats others, especially women, with little respect. In one scene, Dorothy simply bashes him over the head. "Southwest General is made of people."

Julie Nichols (played by Jessica Lange) assumes the role of the nurse in the soap opera. She is quite attractive, but her femininity overextends itself into passivity. Julie's boyfriend (in the movie, not the soap opera) is the director of the show. He comes across as a condescending jerk who treats women like sex objects. Dorothy can't understand why Julie puts up with this behavior and coaches her on how to fend for herself and become more assertive. Soon, Dorothy and Julie become best friends and soulmates. Julie even brings Dorothy home one weekend to meet her dad. Of course, the old man promptly falls for Dorothy and eventually offers her an engagement ring. But Dorothy (that is, Michael) is falling for Julie. In one scene, Dorothy comes on emotionally to Julie, only to be categorized as a lesbian. This movie really is a soap opera!

The final crisis comes when, because of the show's popularity, Dorothy's contract is extended for another year. Now Michael is panicky over the charade he is playing. Finally, during a scene in the show, Dorothy reveals herself for who she really is—Michael Dorsey.

Julie is totally shocked and crushed by the exposure. She wants nothing more to do with Michael. However, in the final scene in the movie, Michael waits outside the stage door as Julie appears. He pleads for understanding as they walk together down the street, explaining that he didn't want to hurt anyone. He just did it for the money. Finally, Julie says that Dorothy "taught me how to stand up for myself. . . . [Dorothy] taught me to stop hiding and be myself. . . . I miss her!"

The movie ends with Michael responding with these classic transformational lines: "You don't have to [miss Dorothy]. She's right here. She misses you. Look, you don't know me from Adam. But I was a better man with you as a woman [as Dorothy] than I ever was as a man with a woman. I just have to learn how to do it without the dress. The hard part's over. We are already good friends."

As they walk away together, Julie asks if she can borrow Dorothy's yellow dress.

Joseph Jaworski and Synchronicity

The world shattered for Joseph Jaworski when he was 41 years old. Returning home one evening, out of the blue his wife confronted him with the announcement, "Joe, I want a divorce. There's somebody else I love."[6]

Joe is the son of Leon Jaworski, the special prosecutor of the infamous Watergate scandal. Like his father, he had become a very successful attorney with all the trappings of success. He was a partner with a prestigious law firm specializing in domestic and international litigation. With some of his college buddies, he invested in businesses on the side and made fabulous returns on his money.

Like many highly paid professionals, Joe lived a picture-book life in a large home, surrounded by all the material things one could desire. He traveled to exotic places, partied hard with his buddies, and in his book *Synchronicity* implies having and being with girlfriends.

Jaworski suggests that what he learned about Watergate from his father caused him to reexamine his personal life's path. Undoubtedly, that was the beginning of a new journey for him, but perhaps the impact of his divorce was even more life fracturing. He was devastated by his wife's announcement and the ensuing separation. For several months thereafter, it appears that he began to embrace the feminine side of his personality. Joe speaks of becoming receptive to and expressing his feelings. In his book, he describes the vital need "to be" as well as "to do," especially to being receptive as one searches for a true vocational calling. He speaks about giving up control and allowing life to flow through him. In short, Joe embraced his feminine opposite and learned how to dance with her. With much depth and humility, the remainder of Joe's book describes the amazing events of his life leading to synchronicity and the establishment of the Centre for Generative Leadership.

The word *synchronicity,* coined by Carl Jung, describes those remarkable events when things come together in an almost inconceivable way. People and events can mysteriously weave themselves into a common thread. In terms of the individual, one senses involvement in an event as though it were meant to be, a kind of destiny. With respect to groups, a diverse body of individuals become aligned to a common purpose. This leads to a discussion of soul and community.

References

[1] T. S. Eliot, *Four Quartets* (New York: Harcourt, Brace & World, 1943), p. 39.

[2] Edward O. Wilson, *The Diversity of Life* (Cambridge, Mass.: The Belknap Press of Harvard University Press, 1992), p. 35.

[3] Tom Chappell, *The Soul of a Business* (New York: Bantam Books, 1993), p. 129.

[4] Michael Ray and Rochele Myers, *Creativity in Business* (New York: Doubleday, 1989), p. 91.

[5] Rainer Maria Rilke, *Letters to a Young Poet* (New York: Vintage Books, 1984), pp. 34–35.

[6] Joseph Jaworski, *Synchronicity* (San Francisco: Berrett-Koehler Publishers, 1996), p. 32.

CHAPTER EIGHT

Soul and Community

*"In a culture where more than 75 percent
of the population do not know their neighbors,
people are starving for connectedness."*[1]

—Joel and Michelle Levey

*N*ature serves as a wonderful teacher of community. For example, did you know that geese—those beautiful Vs cutting through the sky—fly 70 percent faster than a single goose?[2]

HIGH-FLYING GEESE

*G*eese, like all birds, are able to fly because they have open-ended lungs. Most air-breathing animals, like humans, have lungs that are basically enclosed sacs. We draw the air in to cleanse the blood and then exhale it. But in birds, the air passes right through the lungs to a system of air sacs extending throughout the body, including the larger bones. This indicates how an otherwise earthbound creature remains buoyant in both air and water. When geese fly, they are upheld by the air around them but also by the air within them.

In addition to flying faster in a V-shaped community, geese take turns sharing the lead. But at the same time, the lead goose in the formation actually is not doing any more work than the rest. Apparently, there is an aerodynamic principle at work called "upwash," which means that the beating of all those wings creates a current of air that pushes the whole formation along. Even the goose flying in "point" position is lifted up and propelled forward, creating an amazing synergy. Because of this phenomenon, flocks of geese have been known to travel as many as 1,700 miles in two days. No goose flying solo could survive such a trip.[3]

High-flying geese are an excellent example of soul in community, exhibiting some of the key characteristics of soulful communities. First, they obviously have a *shared vision:* they migrate twice a year to a particular destination. Second, they display a high level of *trust and support* for each other: the symmetry of high-flying geese is a beauty to behold. Third, they exhibit *shared leadership* as different members of the flock take to the point.

Finally, geese *care* for one another in times of difficulty and crisis. It sometimes seems that nature's code translates into the survival of the fittest in an impersonal and uncaring manner. But for geese at least, it's different. Not only do they mate for life, but they enjoy an elaborate system of caring in their relationships. When a wounded goose falls to earth, the others in the gaggle come down with it. They wait for the stricken bird to recover or die, sometimes at great cost and risk to themselves from other animals and from hunters. Geese represent a remarkable example of a caring, soulful community.

In *Identity,* Barnhouse raises the question, "Who am I, naked and alone in a white room?"[4] The literal answer she gives: nobody. She suggests that identity (and individuality) are experienced only in terms of background and community. Therefore, reclaiming soul in health care must address a deep human need for community and friendships. We social creatures need each other not only for company but also for meaning in our lives. Considering that most of us spend half or more of our waking hours at work, the need to participate in a community as we work becomes even more acute.

The development of community and friendships at work broadens perspective. Each person brings a sphere of skills, experiences, and personality characteristics that makes the group greater than the sum of its parts. Friendships in particular contribute to the soul and productivity of an organization; without them, the organization is feeble and lifeless. According to Chappell, the enhancement of community and friendship is an alternative to the soulless, harsh, bottom-line mentality of many American businesses.

From a patient's perspective, the energy sensed from a feeling that everyone is part of the same team whose objective is healing "me" is important in the caring prescription. Consider the diminishing confidence in overall care when patients see employees treating each other with a lack of trust and respect.

All of the qualities used to describe high-flying geese also find expression in true human communities, whether found in health care or elsewhere. As described in the previous three chapters, community also thrives when people are treated as individuals, when diversity is pursued, and when employees are placed in jobs suitable to their vocational gifts.

TYPES OF RELATIONSHIPS IN ORGANIZATIONS

In The Community of the Future, Gifford Pinchot describes three types of relationships in social systems: (1) relationships based on power, in which those in positions of authority and power dictate the behaviors of subordinates; (2) relationships based on voluntary exchange, as in trading or buying; and (3) relationships that hinge on the giving of gifts to each other.[5]

Obviously many organizations, and especially those engaged in a business, operate, at least in part, on command and control. Someone must provide leadership, and it is hoped this leadership uses power humanely and with consideration of all the stakeholders. Until recently, most business and health care structures were organized into hierarchies, with one person at the top making strategic decisions. Of course, today many innovative and progressive organizations find it more fruitful to organize around tasks in functional units, indicated in "hub and spoke" structures with power and authority delegated to groups according to their experience, knowledge, and skills.

Still, many organizations function according to apotheosis, meaning the glorification of the heroic ego, the adoration of power and competitiveness. In health care, the heroic ego may sometimes find expression in the exaltation of the all-knowing, teaching, professional doctor. Because of the information explosion, however, few organizations will survive in a heroic ego kind of structure. True, effective, community-oriented organizations are more like a circle with shared gifts and leadership—like high-flying geese, even though geese fly in a V and not a circle.

Apotheosis and the Dreadful Fate of Dr. Semmelweis

What happened to Dr. Ignaz Semmelweis is a sad but true story about the negative effects of apotheosis. In 1846 Dr. Semmelweis was appointed first assistant of the obstetrical clinic at Vienna's General Hospital. The ward he oversaw had two divisions; patients in one division were cared for by physicians, whereas midwives performed all deliveries in the second group. What baffled virtually everyone was the fact that the mortality rate among mothers and babies was nearly 15 percent in the division served by the physicians and only about 3 percent in the section served by midwives.

In those days, physicians performed autopsies as a matter of routine to further understand the nature of human disease. They would wipe their bloody hands on their aprons; in fact, doctors wearing their bloody smocks while making hospital rounds had become a kind of status symbol of their profession.

The tragic death of his mentor and friend, Dr. Jakob Kolletschka, led Dr. Semmelweis to solve the puzzle of the differing mortality rates. Dr. Kolletschka accidentally punctured his finger while performing an autopsy and died from an infection. Dr. Semmelweis theorized from this that the physicians themselves and their bloody hands were causing the high mortality rate in their division. He instituted a rigid hand-washing protocol among the midwives in the other division and the mortality rate fell immediately to near zero. His message was simple: doctors need to wash their hands and remove bloody aprons before seeing patients.

Dr. Semmelweis lost his job at the clinic a year later. It seems that a bloody smock or apron was a visible sign of one's professional importance. Doctors were not about to relinquish a symbol of their status just because some "crackpot" had evidence that hand washing could save lives. Apotheosis, an unbending pride and arrogance, drove Dr. Semmelweis from his profession, and he finally died a lonely death in an insane asylum.

Authority, power, and status are inevitable human attributes to be used for better or worse. The challenge is to apply them with care and good judgment.

All of us can relate to the second type of relationship identified by Pinchot that is based on trading or buying. It is as ancient as civilization itself. Buying in particular is the engine driving our economy. It finds its best expression in a true democracy, one seeking to give everyone an equal opportunity to accumulate wealth and purchasing power.

Next we describe the third characteristic of social systems identified by Pinchot that offers ways of enhancing soul in community.

Gift Giving

The oldest and most universal of social systems is based on the gift economy. It is prevalent everywhere, an a priori function, although few people appear to view it consciously. The earth is a gift.

Life is certainly a gift. The human body functions as a system of organs providing services to each other, like the lungs giving oxygen to the blood.

Although we may be unaware of it, gift giving is in our genes. Hyde reminds us that in the earliest hunter-gatherer societies, status was a function of who killed or gathered food for the entire group.[6] Hyde also reminds us of the Native American, whose practice of passing the peace pipe represents the concept of circular gift giving. The peace pipe continually circulating among the people served as a symbol of communal sharing. Coined by early English settlers, the term "Indian giver" is a misinterpretation of what really was happening.

Another example comes from a practice of Northwest Native Americans. At the raising of a totem, participants would give away all of their worldly possessions. The ceremony surrounding this gift giving highlighted the reality that we come into this world with nothing and we will leave with nothing. Also, to this day some Japanese practice a similar ritual: if you admire something in a Japanese home and touch it, your host may give it to you.

In America we could easily question how much gift giving takes place from the heart as opposed to obligation. We could also ask how much health care is a gift from the heart versus a legislated mandate. For example, how many services are provided to the indigent within the boundaries of available financial resources as opposed to simply fulfilling state-mandated obligations?

Gift giving often finds its expression in the ritual surrounding the sharing of food. It is often joked that hospital staff will eat anything not nailed down. We may laugh, but there are frequent opportunities in various departments or nursing units for staff to share special homemade dishes—yet another example of how humans function in community. The ritual of sharing food is central to both happy and sad occasions.

One medium-sized hospital found itself one year facing budgetary problems. Previously, the hospital had served an elaborate employee dinner each year at Christmas. The senior management team understood the importance of the dinner, but it believed it couldn't justify the expense in light of anticipated cutbacks. Understanding the dilemma, an employee group designed an alternative event, but one that would honor the community's being together at the holiday season. First, the holiday event theme focused on employees being a family and was called "Home for Christmas." Each department, from housekeeping to administration, was invited to hold an open house where employees brought foods prepared from favorite recipes. Some employees played musical instruments and entertained during their open house.

In addition, employees were invited to join a hospital caroling group that sang throughout the halls, both day and evening shifts. The director of housekeeping was a talented guitarist and accompanied them. This family approach was enormously successful, resulting in a heightened sense of community, and patients and visitors were touched by the efforts.

One department manager tells the story of another kind of community event she experienced while working for a former employer. In this particular department, names of employees were drawn for pen pals. Participation was not mandatory, but few employees chose not to participate. During the year, people would do special things, bring surprise gifts, send cards, or in other ways simply perk up the day for their special pen pal. Secrecy was well maintained. At the end of the year, each pen pal was identified during the department's employee dinner.

During the career assessment process, Jim leads his clients through a program to identify key, satisfying skills. They represent gifts so close and vital to each client that they simply can't remain unused and not given to others. Even money, ultimately, is not the motivating factor in using such passionate skills as a way of giving to others.

One nurse reports that the highlight of her career so far has been volunteering a month of health care service to the people of Haiti. She reports that providing this service is for the sheer joy of helping people unable to obtain adequate nursing in other ways. Yet she refuses to consider them poor. "Even in the midst of their physical poverty, I found these people to be filled with joy and spirit. I received much more than I gave them during my visit."

Dr. Ruth Barnhouse, a psychiatrist and Episcopal priest, often states during lectures and workshops that people do far more good than bad. If this were not true, the human species would have become extinct long ago. We hear and read so much in the news about shootings, riots, and the like that we forget about the enormous good that ordinary people do on a daily basis. We are not simply self-serving creatures. Take a trip to the airport or on an airplane and ask for assistance of some kind, and not just from the paid staff. Count the number of people who extend themselves to help you.

BUILDING ON THE GOOD

*E*arlier we mentioned a simple technique called appreciative inquiry (AI), which involves seeking out and advancing life-giving, community-building forces already existing in an organization. We can find health in even the sickest organizations. Indeed, looking for good in the midst of an evil environment produces such events as that depicted in the movie *Schindler's List.*

The basic process of AI is not to see organizations as problems to be solved as much as it is to search for the best of what is. We aren't suggesting that an organization deny or suppress its problems or its shadow. On the contrary, when people promote the good while at the same time acknowledging complexity, they can face problems without being overwhelmed by them. The traditional problem-solving approach to instituting change often stems from the assumption that the organization is a machine. Amplifying the best of what is tends to give the group an organic, soulful web of connectedness.[7]

An appreciative inquiry project essentially involves three phases. The first is data gathering, usually done in nontraditional ways. Researchers and linear thinkers tend to gather data in abstract forms, but in AI, information is generally gathered through stories. Employees are asked to share peak experiences related to the particular topic at hand—their

> *"One thing may be immutable and unchanging—the need to share stories that inspire, teach, and guide new and old members of the organization."*[8]
>
> —Richard Stone
>
>

best individual or team experiences. Storytelling (see chapter 5) is one of the best means of experiencing soul. People love to tell soul stories.

An AI intervention could involve a study of the organization as a whole, although this is quite time-consuming. More manageable examinations could focus on specific issues like teamwork, leadership, or customer/patient satisfaction. Although not specifically labeled appreciative inquiry, many employee activities are based to some degree on AI, thus supporting that which is right in organizations. Employee activities also help in building relationships and connectedness within the organization and across department lines.

One hospital CEO found his new hospital sadly lacking in relationships and connectedness. When he took over, staff morale was low and attrition high. He resolved to reverse this trend. As a result, a new nonmanagerial employee "spirit" group was formed across department lines. The group's task was to promote fun and to recognize employees for their hard work and contribution to the success of the hospital. A new employee recognition program was instigated at about the same time.

Over time, the spirit group became the central focus for employee activities, planning special holiday events and other celebrations. Each Valentine's Day, the group sold inexpensive mementos that employees could send to anyone in the hospital, and that were delivered by a member of the spirit committee. Frequently, valentines were sent by individuals or a department to another person or department in appreciation for help or support at a particular time. A fun activity, it heightened respect and reinforced relationships.

The second step in the process of AI is gaining understanding and insight from the information gathered. This can be somewhat tedious, especially for people who are not oriented toward analyzing data. Again, however, when the information to be examined is in the form of personal stories, the task is significantly enlivened. In addition, the data are personalized because, as all the stories are positive, the actual name of the storyteller can be shared. Storytelling creates energy around issues and promotes even more discussion.

The final step in the process amplifies the information gathered. This step is the envisioning process, determining how the group can move forward and build on examples of superior performance. It brings into play one of the most powerful energies available to humans, which is the use of the imagination.

Imagination nourishes the soul; without it we become detached from soul. "I am indeed convinced," said Carl Jung, "that creative imagination is the only primordial phenomenon accessible to us, the real Ground of the psyche, the only immediate reality. Therefore I speak of *esse in anima* [being in the soul], the only form of being that we can experience directly."[9]

Imagination is not simply child's play, although children have a natural gift of imagination and we would do well to reclaim that gift as adults. The last time Jim visited the dentist, he overheard a conversation with a four-year-old boy who was getting his teeth cleaned for the first time. The technician introduced the vacuum device for removing water and saliva from the mouth as Mr. Thirsty. Now, that's imagination!

Imagination emerges from facts, substance, and experience. It involves imaging and reimaging. For example, we could experience or simply picture an operating room team functioning together with precision, each person performing a function in sync with all the others, each knowing precisely who does what. We could build on this image and apply it to an entire health care community, creating a new vision of "how we operate around here." In fact, this is exactly how AI works. You could interview the

> *"Imagination is more important than knowledge."*
>
> —Albert Einstein

staff of an operating room, soliciting stories of peak experiences. In some respects, such stories could serve as a model for the entire organization.

The next example shows how AI is used in health care. A key strength of one small hospital is its focus on delivering a level of patient-centered care that has differentiated it from other hospitals in the area. Not content with the hospital's already high level of service, employees are forming an interdepartmental employee team to examine all of their patient service opportunities and highlight those they do particularly well. Then they will imagine how these might be strengthened, working to increase the already excellent patient satisfaction reports they receive. Not only will this approach benefit their patients, but it will continue to differentiate them in the marketplace.

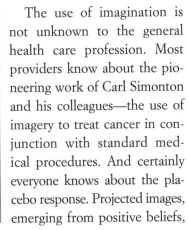

"Imagination is not divorced from the facts; it is a way of illuminating the facts. . . . It enables men [and women] to construct an intellectual vision of a new world."[10]

—Alfred North Whitehead

The use of imagination is not unknown to the general health care profession. Most providers know about the pioneering work of Carl Simonton and his colleagues—the use of imagery to treat cancer in conjunction with standard medical procedures. And certainly everyone knows about the placebo response. Projected images, emerging from positive beliefs, somehow kindle a healing response.

Active imagination can serve as a powerful tool for enhancing soul in an organization, bringing out the best in people and building on it.

BUILDING ON RESPECT

Community in large part is built on respect. We traditionally involve ourselves in groups or organizations in which we feel respected and trusted. Otherwise, we flounder in a sea alone.

In one city several community health agencies became affiliated under one umbrella agency. Although each of the entities remained separate, their affiliated relationship offered a unified presence and reduced their individual operating expenses. All the agencies moved into one building and shared an administrative staff and board of directors. It was one of the earliest affiliation models in this particular city.

On the surface, such an organizational model offered multiple benefits to each of its component groups. Each member agency had its own separate part of the building but shared common conference rooms and kitchen areas. The challenge for the larger group was to build trustful and respectful relationships to replace the previous limited contact. Although some organized effort was made by management to build one community, it was the employees who basically fostered the feeling of one community. Community began with the respect that the employees had for each other's professional expertise and skills. They were not hesitant to ask for advice about some of the clients they served, occasionally referring them to others in their group. Employees often brought lunch to work, eating together in one of the common areas. Friendships developed along with a real feeling of community, even though technically each of the agencies remained separate.

The issue of respect cannot be overemphasized. It is respect that allows people to work together in community. One new CEO of a large hospital replaced a man who was admired and known for the respect he gave his employees. The new CEO made no effort to learn about his administrative team as individuals, nor did he make an effort to retain the feeling of community that previously existed. It soon became obvious that he respected only those individuals who brought business to the hospital, particularly certain members of the medical staff. It was not unusual for him to stand in the middle of the hall and yell for one of his staff, and he frequently called staff out of meetings. Such lack of respect created a fractured community. Survival under the new CEO became the most important objective for the administrative staff, and a one-upmanship mentality developed while employees continually worked on keeping in the CEO's good graces.

ESTABLISHING AND MAINTAINING TRUST

Respect is a cornerstone for building and maintaining trust. A lack of trust almost always means that we are fearful of not being treated with dignity and fairness.

Trust is an elemental need. If a child cannot trust his or her parents to provide food, shelter, and affection, severe neurosis soon develops. Emotional wounds often remain throughout the lifetime of such a child. In a similar manner, love, in the form of emotional attraction, is not the primary foundation on which to build a marriage. A marriage "made in heaven" forms itself on the basis of respect and trust.

Trust results in honesty, openness, connectedness, and an increased desire to contribute to the organization. It encourages people to be authentic with each other. A high level of trust reflects the organization's ability to bring to the surface differences in values and opinions and to deal with them in constructive ways. On the other hand, a low level of trust results in hostility, power struggles, alienation, diminished levels of productivity, and, ultimately, turnover.

A major Fortune 500 company announced a comprehensive reorganization in the early 1990s. Roughly 30 percent of the workforce, almost 4,500 employees, opted to accept either an early retirement package or voluntary severance. A lack of trust contributed at least partially to this amazing response; the number of employees opting to leave was probably more than double what senior management had estimated. Granted, the severance package was extremely generous; however, employees at the peak of their careers, with 10 to 20 years of service, opted out. In an organization blessed with a high level of trust, this undoubtedly wouldn't have happened.

This company's respect for the human effects of the reorganization was also lacking. Financial planning programs were held for all those deciding to accept early retirement; however, no effort was made to help employees through the emotional trauma of making life-changing decisions. The reorganization lacked compassion, at least in the eyes of many employees. Nurturing community is essential in the soulful organization. Doing their jobs well is almost impossible for employees without a community's shared gifts—their trust and respect for each other.

INDIVIDUAL IN COMMUNITY VERSUS INDIVIDUALISM

*I*n any soul-enhancing group—a business, health care organization, or society in general—community and individuality must be kept in a kind of paradoxical balance.[11] Figure 8-1 depicts the needs, rights, privileges, and duties of the individual on the one side and those of the community on the other. A tension exists between the two sides, and, of course, the question is how to balance them.

Balance is absolutely imperative. People are in trouble either as individuals, groups, or nations if there is imbalance in either direction. For example, if we attempt to function entirely as individuals on our own, in the extreme we would go insane. Sensory deprivation experiments have proved that if all stimuli are withdrawn from an individual, in a matter of hours that person will begin to hallucinate. We need input from other people in order to survive. It is indisputable that "no man is an island unto himself."

On the other hand, if we only define ourselves in terms of our background, parents, and community without a conscious sense of personal uniqueness, we enjoy little or no sense of individuality. Such a person engages only in herd mentality. In order to enjoy true, mature personhood, there must be a balance between being separate from others and being connected to them.

FIGURE 8-1

Balancing Individuality and Community

Needs		*Needs*
Rights		*Rights*
Privileges		*Privileges*
Duties		*Duties*
Individual		**Community**

Our culture leans heavily on the side of personal freedom and rugged individualism as opposed to being a responsible person in a community. More than sufficient evidence exists that American culture is overbalanced on the side of individualism. We evaluate people on the basis of how well they can stand on their own two feet. Our culture expects children to become self-reliant at a very young age and begin competing with each other. The inference is that one must compete with others to have personal needs and desires met. Even though all of us are inadequate in one form or another, our society views inadequacy as a character flaw. This can be linked to the intense loneliness in our culture that results in all kinds of addictions and abuse.

On the other hand, many cultures with significant problems are overbalanced on the side of community. Many developing Eastern cultures are grounded in the values of the collective, in which individuals are expected to submerge their own needs, rights, privileges, and duties in favor of the group. Americans often view this as totalitarian and damaging to individual liberty, but we don't realize how these societies recoil in equal horror at our culture, viewing it as being one of unchecked, personal selfishness.

Democracy in its truest form stands in the middle, protecting the rights of the individual while promoting the needs of the community, including the sustenance of the physical environment. Authentic democracy serves us well as a form of soulful governance. In a democratic society, freedom and responsibility become two sides of the same coin. You can't have one without the other. Freedom without responsibility results in license to do as you please and ends in chaos. A person who opts for freedom without responsibility is really not free but rather is a prisoner of impulses.

On the other hand, if one opts only for responsibility, it leads to rigidity and a kind of judgmental moralism. Responsibility without freedom stifles play, imagination, creativity, and spontaneity. Soul thrives in an environment where people live freely with responsibility. It is where both individuality and community are cherished.

References

1 Joel Levey and Michelle Levey, "Chaos to Community at Work," in *Community Building in Business,* ed. Kazimerz Gozdz (San Francisco: New Leaders Press, 1995), p. 105.

2 Browne Barr, *High-Flying Geese* (New York: Seabury Press, 1973).

3 We are indebted to the Rev. Kathlyn James, United Methodist minister, for this information along with other insights presented in this chapter.

4 Ruth Tiffany Barnhouse, *Identity* (Philadelphia: Westminister Press, 1984), p. 17.

5 Frances Hesselbein, Marshall Goldsmith, and Richard Beckhard, eds., Peter F. Drucker Foundation, *The Community of the Future* (San Francisco: Jossey-Bass Publishers, 1998).

6 Lewis Hyde, *The Gift, Imagination and the Erotic Life of Property* (New York: Vintage Books, 1979).

7 Sue Annis Hammond, *The Thin Book of Appreciative Inquiry* (Plano, Tex.: Kodiak Consulting, 1996).

8 Richard Stone, "The Self-Knowing Organization," *StoryWork Institute Newsletter* (winter/spring, 1998): 5.

9 C. G. Jung, *Letters,* vol. 1, eds. G. Adler and A. Jaffe, trans. R. F. C. Hull (Princeton, N.J.: Princeton University Press, 1973), p. 60.

10 Alfred North Whitehead, *The Aims of Education and Other Essays* (New York: Macmillan Co., 1929), p. 139.

11 We are endebted to Ruth Tiffany Barnhouse, MD, MDiv, for the majority of the material in this section. It was presented at a lecture at Southern Methodist University's Perkins School of Theology in 1984. More information on balance between individuality and community can be found in her book *Identity,* note 4.

CHAPTER NINE

Applications of Soul in Organizations

*"A lot of our celebrations are spontaneous. . . .
It has to be an event that praises the goodness
of soul and brings out the idealism
and the altruism of people."*[1]
—Herb Kelleher, CEO, Southwest Airlines

A significant number of U.S. corporations and health care organizations are consciously promoting soul. We begin this chapter with perhaps the best example of a corporation advancing soul in the non–health care field, followed by additional illustrations.

NON–HEALTH CARE EXAMPLES

Southwest Airlines

We first witnessed the soul of Southwest Airlines during an airplane trip in Texas. Leaving the plane and walking down the airport hallway, we were drawn to a large display of pictures in which airline employees were wearing all kinds of crazy outfits and balloons were clinging to the ceiling. And there was CEO Herb

Kelleher propped on a custom Harley-Davidson motorcycle, given to him by some of the employees.

The colorful story of Southwest's birth is vividly reported by Kevin and Jackie Freiberg in *Nuts!*.[2] They chronicle the incredibly difficult David and Goliath battles fought over a four-year period before the first airplane flew on June 18, 1971.

We define culture as "the way we operate around here," and *Nuts!* truly documents the airline's soulful corporate culture. A soulful business culture grounds itself in the values implicit in the Freibergs' book: energy, vitality, connectedness, depth of spirit, and mutual caring at all levels of the organization. It rests on the four pillars of individuality, career satisfaction, diversity, and community.

Southwest Airlines adds a fifth quality of soul—fun! "We feel this fun atmosphere builds a strong sense of community. It also counterbalances the stress of hard work and competition," says Elizabeth Sartain.[3] The idea of having fun at work originally surfaced because, during the 1970s, the airline had extremely limited funds for marketing. So employees were asked to come up with resourceful ways to entertain their customers and make them laugh. One flight attendant actually hid in a luggage bin; when a customer opened the bin, she handed him a soft drink.

Not only is having fun a corporate value, but in *Nuts!* the Freibergs' identify 12 other dominant values that drive the company. Core values particularly related to soul include family and love.

"A family atmosphere simply means . . . that you are sincerely interested in everyone . . . and can forgive some eccentricities," says Kelleher.[4] And family is not limited to the immediate workforce but also includes the extended family. Employees periodically bring their children to work, and spouses appear at important company events.

Southwest encourages employees to care for others—fellow employees and customers—in a loving manner. This is affirmed by treating people with dignity and extending care into the greater community through service projects. Love is not simply a mushy concept at Southwest but reflects the nature of true love, which is an act of giving (the gift economy). *Nuts!* dedicates an entire chapter to gift giving, offering many examples. Did you know that Southwest transported volunteers to the Oklahoma City bombing disaster site at no charge?

Southwest Airlines is a superb example of how enhancing soul contributes to the bottom line. In 1991 Southwest transported 2,318 passengers per employee as compared with an industry average of 848. In the same year it had the fewest number of employees per aircraft. The airline's turnover rate of employees is the lowest in the industry. From 1972 through 1992, Southwest had the highest percentage return of all airline stocks.

Tom's of Maine

Tom Chappell founded Tom's of Maine, a firm manufacturing and selling environmentally safe health care products, such as toothpaste. He based his company on the concept that you could make a product that was good for the environment as well as for people.[5] He also embraced the belief that there is nothing wrong with making a profit so long as it is done ethically and responsibly.

As the company grew, however, with MBAs and people from other industries brought in, Chappell discovered that the value system of the firm began moving in the wrong direction. As often happens during expansion, it experienced a shrinking of its original vision, and Chappell became disenchanted by the company's movement toward a bottom-line mentality.

About this time, Chappell attended an event at Harvard Divinity School designed to communicate the nature of an institution's mission. Deeply impressed, he shortly thereafter enrolled in the school as a special student and spent four years there while working half-time at his business in Maine. He began to use his business as a laboratory for what he was learning in theology and philosophy classes. Some of the most significant principles he applied to business came from Martin Buber's description of "I" and "Thou" and from Jonathan Edwards's concept of "being in relation." These principles follow closely the qualities of soul we've described. For Chappell, being in relation came to mean valuing one's relationships with employees, customers, vendors, the environment, one's community, and the government. Most business organizations affect these entities and are influenced by them.

In addition, Buber has suggested that there are two attitudes by which we perceive the world and act on it. The first perception is that we are in relation to the environment (human beings, trees, and so on) as objects ("I-It" relationship), as means to accomplish a higher purpose such as profit. However, the other type of attitude suggests an "I-Thou" relationship, which is to stand before an entity with respect and awe. It develops, in part, as a natural consequence of adopting a soulful approach to the universe. It also comes from an understanding that everything is connected and alive and has value and worth in and of itself.

Chappell pondered the possibility of adopting this second, sacred attitude in a business setting, while at the same time being productive and profitable. For him it seemed possible to bring the two attitudes together, integrating the world of "I-Thou" with the perception of "I-It" to bring about the best of productivity with the best of respect.

He brought his board members and staff together to study these concepts. They engaged in a creative process of discussing who they were as a company. The ideas were formulated into a statement of corporate beliefs and mission.[6] Tom's of Maine now incorporates both a belief in the inherent worth and dignity of human beings and an understanding that one can be financially successful while behaving in a responsible manner.

Over a period of time, the belief and mission statements became an operational force. Like our use of the circle as a metaphor for soul, Tom's of Maine employs the circle as a metaphor for how it operates. It represents a way of each employee being equal in relation to every other. All people concerned about a particular problem or having influence on the introduction of a new product are brought together. A dialogue ensues, generating as many ideas as possible around the issue. Diversity in particular is sought for gaining a variety of perspectives. Within the circle, employees feel comfortable in sharing, listening, playing, and using their imaginations. New products and services often emerge through this process, largely because of a high level of trust. Trust springs from the attitude that each person is just as worthy as everyone else, regardless of position within the firm.

The 75-plus employees of Tom's of Maine reflect the diversity of mainstream America. Their commitment to diversity is operational and intentional. When recruiting talent through employment firms, headhunters are instructed to submit a list of diverse candidates. This commitment to diversity cascades throughout all levels of recruiting activity.

The opposite of diversity is sameness. Sameness squelches creativity. It stifles soul in the sense of limiting an organization to a one-dimensional view of business and the marketplace. To avoid sameness, Tom's of Maine promotes complexity in the organization, not only in terms of its employees, but also as a total business strategy. It influences marketing strategy. "We believe in a diversity of products supporting one common brand—Tom's of Maine— and we believe this makes Tom's increasingly excellent as a company."[7] Tom's has more varieties of toothpaste than Proctor & Gamble, including Cinnamint with Propolis & Myrrh, Children's Orange, and Silly Strawberry.

Like Southwest Airlines, the company incorporates a form of human association very much in the forefront of discussion and concern in our culture—the family. "At Tom's of Maine, we want to see all sides of every person working together; we want to know one another as warehouse worker/father/husband, as vice-president/ wife/mother/citizen."[8] Therefore, periodic "celebration breaks" are held, gatherings designed for storytelling and sharing what is happening in the lives of the employees. The company established summer lifestyle hours, fitting in 40 hours of work from Monday until noon on Friday, in response to employees' valuing lifestyle integration along with earning a wage. The company also offers parenting leaves whereby fathers as well as mothers have an opportunity to spend a month or so bonding with newborn children. Tom's of Maine was recognized by *Working Mother* for three consecutive years as one of the 100 best companies for working mothers.

This commitment to community extends beyond the immediate workforce. The company's mission includes addressing community concerns in Maine and around the world. The company tithes, giving 10 percent of its pretax profits to various organizations. For example, in 1996 it committed $100,000 to support the work of the Rainforest Alliance, a not-for-profit organization working to preserve the world's endangered tropical forests. Employees are also encouraged to use 5 percent of their paid worktime for volunteer activities of their choosing.

It is through the activities described above that Tom's of Maine integrates the bottom-line mentality with soul, the masculine with the feminine, and doing with being. And it pays off. By 1996 it had garnered 5 percent of many of the major urban markets, competing with giants like Proctor and Gamble—no small feat in such a competitive world,[9] and it has been growing consistently by 20 percent from 1993 to the present.

Washington Mutual Bank

On a sparkling day in September 1995, the plane lifted quickly, circling over the L-shaped Puget Sound. Heading southwest, off to the left we viewed the majestic, snow-blanketed peak of Mt. Rainier as we were returning from a splendid autumn week visiting Jim's son and his family. We're not sure who started the conversation, but one of us said, "Let's move." The other replied, "Why not? There's little to keep us in Dallas." "What about the rain?" "Well, it's a matter of give and take. What about the summer heat in Texas?"

Workwise, neither of us had many constraints. After 20 years, Jim had accepted an early retirement package from a utility company and currently was contracting as a career and outplacement consultant. Linda's business was marketing and communications services. We decided to move as soon as one of us found work in Seattle, so we began the research and networking process.

We subscribed to the Sunday edition of the *Seattle Times* and in November Jim came across an employment ad for a career planning consultant position with Washington Mutual Bank. He said he didn't want to work for a large corporation again but decided to research the bank anyway. Soon he discovered that the bank was not your usual organization. It had an interesting value system and seemed to "walk the talk." One networking contact said that, except for the low wage scale typically associated with financial institutions, employees were quite loyal and turnover was low. So Jim sent his résumé and application, not expecting any response because Seattle is quite a distance from Dallas.

Surprisingly, however, he received a fax announcing that the human resources manager would be calling him one evening for an interview. What an unusual interview it was, following what he considered an odd format. Jim had taught interviewing skills to many job searchers, but this was a new experience. The questions fell into a simple model, later revealed as "situation . . . action . . . result." "Has your manager ever asked you to do something you didn't think was ethical? How did you respond? What was the result?"

Washington Mutual uses a formal interviewing process called Targeted Selection® developed by Development Dimensions

International. Not only is it used to find the right people for the right job, but also questions can be tailored to determine whether a candidate fits the organization's unique culture.

Washington Mutual prides itself on its high ethical standards. Usually during the first week of employment, people attend an orientation program designed to tell the company's story and communicate its corporate values. Employees, as well as customers, are valued and treated with dignity. In return, they are expected to operate with the highest standards of honesty and integrity. Cooperation, trust, and shared objectives underline the importance of teamwork.

As for the four qualities of soul, the company commits itself to diversity. Jim was 59 years old when he applied for the job, not believing himself to be a viable candidate because of his age. Like many banks, more than 60 percent of the employees are female. Less common, many of the senior managers and executives are also women.

Within a few months following his hiring, Jim and his immediate peers visited the company's telephone banking service operations (TBS). The place has soul. More than 100 employees are allowed—probably encouraged—to customize their workspace with pictures and symbols expressing individuality. As often as possible, work schedules are structured to accommodate family or educational responsibilities. Within limits, it's dress as you please. TBS also provides customized team building and career assessment for its managers and lead supervisors.

Team building is an excellent vehicle for enhancing all four of the qualities of soul, especially through the use of the Myers-Briggs Type Indicator (MBTI®), which reveals how diverse we are as individuals in applying personal skills to the choice of a career path. And it demonstrates how people can complement one another in a team or during a project.

Washington Mutual has been using the MBTI® throughout its organization as a self-learning instrument and to enhance teamwork. At a series of quarterly meetings, more than 250 financial center assistant managers received feedback regarding styles and strengths. During its annual conference, the commercial division of the bank administered the instrument to more than 200 employees and provided insights on how to sell according to strengths and type. Throughout the Northwest, employee relations field consultants have been trained to utilize the MBTI® in financial and loan centers. (An example of team-building use of the MBTI® in health care is in the appendix.)

As mentioned before, the soul of an organization is enhanced by providing vocational development opportunities. Early in the 1990s, Washington Mutual established career-planning services. Although available to all employees, priority was given to assisting those employees whose jobs were being eliminated. Employees received at least 30 days' notice before termination and were assisted in conducting an internal search for an appropriate job. These efforts received support from a comprehensive job-posting system whose goal was to retain valued workers. In 1996 more than 90 percent of the employees affected by reductions were successful in finding new employment within the company. Unfortunately, that figure fell significantly as the company expanded into new states and many employees were unwilling to relocate.

Mergers and acquisitions challenge the soul and vitality of an organization, and Washington Mutual is no exception. Over a two-year period beginning in 1996, the workforce grew fourfold, from about 5,000 to more than 33,000 employees. The company expanded from banking only in the Northwest to serving 38 states. Such expansion put enormous pressures on employees, overworking some of them to the point of exhaustion. Unless consciously maintained, soul begins to recede and relinquish itself to other priorities during these periods. Nonetheless, as one employee put it, "Everyone seems to be overworked these days. If it's going to happen to you, you may as well work for a nice company."

HEALTH CARE ORGANIZATIONS

*T*here may be other soulful groups, but we chose examples on the basis of our familiarity with their stories. Nor are we suggesting that these organizations have been spared the same challenges faced by all health care groups or that time and money won't be expended on unsuccessful business strategies. However, intentionally investing in employees through training and building a culture based on values and respect allow health care groups to meet the problems created by the surrounding chaos. It is also probable that, even within the soulful organization, 100 percent of all activities won't happen as desired. As Andrew Fallat of Evergreen Community Health Care states, "I'd like to say that every staff and every supervisor has a certain dialogue and certain relationship, but I can't be certain."

Every health care organization differs in personality and in its reflection of its community. Each may have selected different approaches to enhancing soul, but there's a common thread to their stories. In particular, when intentionally creating an organization built on respect, trust, caring relationships, and connecting to the greater whole are key characteristics, and the true test is sustainability.

Harborview Medical Center

"Mother Harborview," as it is often affectionately called, has always opened its arms to people in need from all socioeconomic levels, with a special emphasis on the indigent and underserved. Its mission mandates that all people are taken care of regardless of their ability to pay. As the only Level I trauma center in a four-state area, Harborview serves Washington, Alaska, Montana, and Idaho, covering a land mass equal to one-fourth of the United States. The acuity level of its patients is extraordinarily high, requiring an intensity of effort and expertise far beyond the norm.

A Seattle-based medical center, Harborview is owned by King County, governed by a county-appointed board of trustees, and managed under contract by the University of Washington. Each of the medical center's 2,900 employees works for the university. The combined structure makes for a unique model; as such, its mission specifically mandates service to a wide and diverse population. David E. Jaffe, executive director/CEO, notes that employees choose to work at Harborview because of their unwavering commitment to the hospital's mission and the desire to be part of an organization on the cutting edge of medicine. Harborview's mission is at the heart and soul of the organization, and Jaffe suggests the commitment to mission keeps employees there even though many of the patients are more difficult to treat and the pay scale is somewhat lower than at other hospitals. "People are fulfilled by working here," Jaffe says. The employee attrition rate averages 10 percent, well below the national average.

The medical staff is provided by the University of Washington School of Medicine. As the only medical school in the state, it serves Washington and its four surrounding states. Employees have the opportunity of working with faculty who have achieved national prominence in their field. "There is a sense of pride when you get really good at what you do," Jaffe says. He emphasizes that Harborview also prides itself on understanding and being sensitive to the social, economic, and cultural diversity of the people it serves.

Harborview's international medicine clinic treats people from Cambodia, Vietnam, and East Africa. Staff receive training in cultural diversity, and a language bank provides translators for more than 80 languages. In 1996 the hospital received two Safety Net awards from the National Association of Public Hospitals. Community House Calls, an outreach program that sends workers into patients' homes, received a Healthy Communities honorable mention for its care to ethnic and refugee communities in Seattle. Four other Harborview outreach programs were also part of the award.

Harborview has received national recognition in a number of specialized areas, and Jaffe notes that it is achieving impressive outcomes. For example, the survival rate for brain aneurysms is among the highest in the nation. In addition, orthopedic residents from across the country, including those from prestigious New York medical schools, rotate through Harborview because of the quality of the program. Harborview also receives over $45 million annually in research grants and some 35 percent of all National Institute of Health's neurosurgery research dollars. Pallidotomy, a new and less invasive procedure for treating Parkinson's disease and other movement disorders, was perfected at Harborview. In addition, the results of current research revolutionizing prehospital trauma care in the field are anticipated within the next couple of years.

"The most powerful ingredient of quality care cannot be commandeered or bought. Neither is it the sole responsibility of doctors and nurses. But caring for one another, every person in a provider organization has the power to contribute to the creation of a healing culture. We are all equal partners in meeting the leadership challenges in health care."[10]

—Irwin M. Rubin

Jaffe considers Harborview's employees its greatest asset. They are supported through ongoing education and training. The medical center's career development program was initiated to nurture employees in career growth. Harborview consistently shares its stories of achievements and highlights employee contributions in internal and external publications, and the importance of each individual to the organization's mission is continually emphasized. Jaffe stresses this message at each new employee orientation. As he says, "Without our employees, there would only be a state-of-the-art shell."

The Institute of Rehabilitation and Research
Located in Houston, Texas, The Institute of Rehabilitation and Research, or TIRR, serves as a teaching hospital for the Baylor School of Medicine and the University of Texas Health Science Center–Houston. Louisa Adelung, president and CEO, considers the soul of her organization integral to the rehabilitation process, which shows up in the interaction between team members and patients. She views health care today as being too driven by the bottom line. For the most part, she believes people gravitate to health care as a profession to make a difference in people's lives, and they become disillusioned when there is too much emphasis on finances. It is like looking at health care from the neck up. Adelung does not dismiss the importance of the bottom line but believes there must be more of a balance between the financial side and the caring side of medicine. The primary context has to be the patient and the patient's outcome. "At TIRR," she adds, "we make money to provide health care as opposed to providing health care to make money."

According to Adelung, TIRR's revitalizing watershed event resulted from a management retreat held a number of years ago. Management staff opened up; old grudges keeping people from working together as a team fell away. With the help of outside resources, the group began learning new communication tools. Adelung likens the experience to "the unleashing of our souls."

The benefits of working together differently filtered down into patient care. The goal of a rehabilitation facility is to help patients become independent. While there had always been an interdisciplinary team representing the usual therapies, in reality they didn't function in an interdisciplinary manner. Specialty team members simply operated in their own silos, setting their goals for the patient and reporting them to the whole group. After the organization's transformation began, they found themselves no longer stuck in that old paradigm; consequently, their effectiveness as a team increased. They began looking at the patient's goals through the patient's eyes, engaging him or her as a partner in healing. Not only did it affect patient satisfaction positively, but it also had a major impact on the bottom line. Lengths of stay were reduced dramatically and outcomes improved significantly.

Other benefits have been traced to a changing emphasis on employee relationships. Historically, TIRR had always been a teaching hospital in the Baylor system. Some six or seven years ago, TIRR management decided that to be successful they needed a connection with the University of Texas. Because the University of Texas Health Science Center didn't have a physical medicine and rehabilitation department, it eventually recruited specialists from Baylor, which split Baylor's department in half and divided the medical school. The tools for effective communication that their physicians learned earlier enabled the two staffs to get past that event. The two chairpersons subsequently formed a joint department combining residency programs and research. The end result was the formation of a premier Physical Medicine and Rehabilitation Program now serving as a role model for other organizations.

In 1997, a new Mission Connect program was launched that joined physicians and research scientists from three medical schools and TIRR's foundation. The TIRR-led consortium's project is committed to reversing the consequences of spinal cord injuries. "The three schools, their enthusiasm to work in a collaborative manner, and the additional strengths of the Texas Medical Center provide the resources necessary to ensure the first-class work the project requires," notes Howard Wolf, TIRR and TIRR Foundation chairman of the boards of trustees.

Adelung believes that the work done is visible within all of the stakeholder groups—including the board, physicians, senior management, and midmanagers. She concedes that additional work is needed with front-line staff but thinks it is at about the 85 percent level. Employees are supported in many ways throughout the organization. Career satisfaction is emphasized, helping employees focus on following their heart's desire. Staff and outsiders alike see TIRR as a very different organization. Patients and institute visitors usually experience more than one hospital before their contact with the TIRR facility. Although they can't define what they feel in so many words, they often comment on how different TIRR seems and how well the staff works together. In 1997 and for the eighth straight year, TIRR was named one of America's best hospitals in a national physician survey reported annually in *U.S. News & World Report.*

Evergreen Community Health Care

According to Evergreen's CEO Andrew Fallat, the meaning of Evergreen's purpose is as important to each staff interaction as it is to patients. He believes that being conscious of caring for the whole person is important, and caring includes staff as well as patients. "If we don't care for each other, where will we get the energy to give to others . . . if we don't replenish ourselves?"

Evergreen is located in the rapidly growing area east of Seattle. Since Fallat took over as CEO, the workforce has grown from 350 to more than 2,000 employees.

A strong believer in leading through building high-quality relationships, Fallat puts caring for each other as the first priority. Senior management began the considerable work of organization transformation in fostering relationships and mutual respect. Although believing Evergreen had a respectful environment, management wanted to determine exactly where the organization stood. To answer this question, managers asked questions: "What would respect mean to people? What would it look like and what would it feel like? How would we know that it was respectful?"

Within a two-week period, meetings for engaging in dialogue with 1,000 employees from all work areas were held. Nurses, housekeepers, pharmacists, and executives met in the same room to explain what respect meant to them. They shared how they performed when they felt they were shown respect and what happened to their ability to perform when they felt they were shown disrespect. Fallat notes that the most powerful analogy came from an employee who liked driving race cars. "When it feels disrespectful and there is tension in the air and I don't know how to deal with it, it is as though I am driving in the fog. But when the pavement is clear and I am respected, I am driving 200 mph down the street. And I'm relaxed. Now when you are driving 200 mph, you do not want to be tense!"

> *"Working together to enrich the health and well-being of every life we touch."*
>
> —Purpose, Evergreen Community Health Care
>
>

Fallat uses this story to show the power of being respected. His colleagues know they are moving at an incredible pace, performing at an unbelievable level, and yet are at ease. "Most folks think of the fast pace [of health care] and tension. The staff are saying that respect allows us to be fast paced and smooth. That type of conversation opened the possibility that we could accomplish great things and enjoy it and be at peace and soulful about it."

Fallat enjoys telling stories to employees to illustrate his ideas. He frequently uses an old English comedy routine about an owner of a bed and breakfast along the English seacoast, whose kitchen and restaurant are separated only by a door. The comedy's central character is always burning food and slapping pots and pans and even his employees. It is always chaos in the kitchen. But when he comes out, he is sweet to the patrons. "Half the joke," says Fallat, "is the way the patrons are responding to this guy who is being obsequious when they know it's just chaos in the background. If we're in chaos with each other, if we're throwing things, or yelling at each other, or creating that kind of tension, do you think the patient doesn't know it when we walk into the room? Do you think the patient doesn't need even more reassurance? So we care for the patient by caring for ourselves."

Evergreen's effort to intentionally enhance relationships began with input from the hospital's obstetricians and maternity nurses, who predicted they could deliver healthier babies more quickly with less pain medication and with shorter lengths of stay if mothers and fathers had confidence in their child's birth plan. The medical team acknowledged that it had to shift from a belief system based on being in charge and having all the answers. It was the family's birth, not the team's. If Evergreen's medical staff could provide high-quality education and were there to prevent unsafe practices, they should then have confidence that the family would make healthy choices. This shift in attitude was accomplished through several years' training and educational programs. As predicted, the level of anesthetics and lengths of stay decreased, patient satisfaction rose, and market share increased. Today Evergreen's Family Maternity Center is acknowledged as outstanding. The center was honored in August 1998 with two *Eastside Parent* magazine's Golden Bootie awards. For the third straight year, Evergreen was recognized by the magazine's readers as the best place to deliver a baby. In addition, the popular Baby–Parent Time support groups were voted the best place to get out of the house with a new baby.

Evergreen's experience with its maternity patients is an example of what a shift in beliefs can do. However, the success didn't transfer to the rest of the organization. It was not until the hospital was considering implementing a hospice program that it became evident that the beginning and end of life shared similar characteristics. By providing the same sort of care for the family and patient before imminent death as the care provided before a birth, the hospital could care for the whole life of a person in which death is just a biological event. Moreover, a similar model is being considered in areas of cardiac, cancer, and pediatric care. Fallat notes, "We are caring for whole people, including their soul, in which we bring a particular element called the medical or physical part. But that only works when it is put in the whole context and we as caregivers can help make the connections." The same holistic philosophy applies to staff, who have learned that when their relationships are solid and well grounded, organizational tasks go much faster.

Senior management believes its efforts provided two benefits to Evergreen staff and patients. First, more thoughtfulness in relating to each other allows staff to see possibilities in problem solving. Second, the emphasis on providing choices encourages growth and well-being. This is equally true for patients and their treatment plans, employees and their careers, and physicians responding to partnering opportunities with the hospital. Today Evergreen has revamped its budgeting process, included the entire staff in strategic planning, and altered its job-interviewing and hiring practices.

Fallat cautions that such organizational work does not prevent problems or layoffs. As the organization responds to new challenges, employee staffing needs too will change. The difference is that Evergreen is committed to being sensitive to what these changes mean to its employees. When several members of the management team realized that appropriate restructuring meant their jobs were unnecessary, they literally designed themselves out of work. As to the downsizing, Fallat says, "We invented our own way; we did it with compassion and caring." Bereavement counselors helped employees understand the grief involved in job loss before it was time to say good-bye. When offered the choice of working through their notice period or leaving, most people chose to stay, working right up to the end. In many organizations, people who are leaving are virtually written off and treated as outsiders. In contrast, Evergreen was determined to treat those leaving as productive and contributing staff members as long as they remained.

Evergreen continues to work on building a trusting environment and a culture built on respect for individuals and their professions. Fallat believes that community occurs when people feel connected. "We are committed to the quality of the professional life of the caregiver. That's what drives us," he says. Such a workplace leads to creative approaches to health care's challenges. Reimbursement limitations typically lead organizations to believe they have no control over outcomes. At Evergreen, employees take control by asking, "What are the possibilities?" As CEO, Fallat believes firmly that what has been started is sustainable in the future and is not dependent on him, "There is a natural flow and evolution, and it's not just my ideas."

Nightime Pediatrics
Nightime Pediatrics Clinics in Salt Lake City, Utah, opened with one clinic some 15 years ago as an after-hours emergency room alternative. In 1997 its five area clinics saw 80,000 children. Developed as a comfortable place for parents to take their children when their pediatrician's office was full or closed, it is open from noon to 7:00 A.M., 365 days a year. It also benefits the Salt Lake City area pediatricians by reducing their long on-call hours.

The facility was custom designed for the children it would serve. Everything speaks to their senses, from the smell to the look and texture of the furnishings. Staff don't wear white lab coats. There is no waiting room as such, but rather, ample treatment rooms facing a central nurses' station. Each room looks like a small living room, equipped with couches and an examining table that appears to be a piece of furniture. A TV and video playing movies and cartoons are in each room. The separate play area for siblings has a video camera broadcasting continually on corner inserts on the TV monitors. Parents feel better about staying with their sick child when they can see what their other children are doing.

The physical environment is not the only unique characteristic of the facility. The clinic was founded on a core set of values and beliefs. "In health care, we are all practitioners. The most important thing is the way we feel about ourselves so that we can help those who don't feel well to feel better. If I can make a difference with just one person who works here, or one child we see, then the effort is worthwhile," says CEO Teresa Lever-Pollary. She views quality as being three-pronged: the medical and technological procedural-based outcomes, fiscal responsibility, and the quality of relationships. She believes it is the latter component that is the soul part of the organization.

Building relationships represents the key to effectiveness. The high level of parental satisfaction reflects the obvious caring among staff as well as the care given to the young patients. The staff's respect for each other allows them to take the approach that even when something new is tried and doesn't work, it becomes an opportunity for learning, not a mistake. Often they may implement the same idea later after a fresh review.

Nightime's original unique clinic model was so successful that growth was rapid. As Lever-Pollary notes, "By the fourth clinic, it was obvious that we were replicating systems, but that something was getting lost. The first [clinic] was built on relationships." It was that piece she came to believe was missing; the rapid growth inhibited relationships. As a result, Lever-Pollary decided that she could no longer support adding new clinics. In spite of the financial losses attributed to growth, she increased the budget for training and employee development. It was her belief that as CEO she had to "walk the talk" of building relationships. With the help of a consultant and committed and supportive management staff, the clinics began rebuilding a culture based on values, emphasizing employee relationships and human growth. Lever-Pollary believes that having such a culture enables employees to solve critical problems and resolve issues.

To those who suggest that rebuilding relationships is soft stuff with little relation to the bottom line, she counters with stories of its financial impact. As recently as two years ago, after another financial loss, the emphasis remained on training and development. Last year, with a half-million dollar turnaround, Nightime began reaping the rewards of investing in its employees.

Lever-Pollary tells the story of how one of her employees equated the new approach to a family's budgeting process. "We have a budget at home and we have money for food and movies. When things get tight, we cut out the movies. Here, some people think training is like the movies. But, in fact, for us it's the food."

Building high-quality relationships has paid off in other ways as well. Its long-term relationship with insurance providers has enabled the group to negotiate an important contract that otherwise would not have been possible. Since Nightime is neither an ER nor a physician

> *"A community occurs when we align our hearts and minds together."*
>
> —Teresa Lever-Pollary, CEO, Nightime Pediatrics Clinics
>
>

practice, appropriate reimbursement rates were difficult to set; the usual coding system doesn't contain charges for such a unique delivery model. Because of Nightime's integrity and the relationship built between its billing and the insurance companies' claims staffs, Lever-Pollary was able to negotiate a fair and equitable rate.

Nightime enjoys considerable patient satisfaction, and area pediatricians are pleased to have the clinics available for their patients. In addition, Nightime experiences a high level of medical staff and employee satisfaction. Many pediatricians and other employees who have left the company return because of their satisfaction with Nightime's environment. The nursing director related one such example. After leaving to take a position with another organization for a $3-per-hour pay increase, one nurse called three months later, asking to return. What she found was that even though nursing functions are basically the same, she missed the Nightime job—the whole experience—and was drawn back. Lever-Pollary reports that organizational structure frequently changes to reflect an employee's career growth; the organization, in fact, celebrates career development.

The interconnectedness of staff and patients has been highlighted in a compilation of short stories contributed by them that aids staff in gaining an increased awareness of their enormous individual contributions. In one of the *Nightime Stories,* an employee tells of her struggle with breast cancer and the support given to her by staff.[11] "Through it all, I never felt that I had to worry about my position. Or how I looked. They wanted me because of my experience, my maturity, and my ability to get the job done, no matter what. . . . Through all these difficult personal trials, my fellow employees have taught me that Nightime is not just about caring for kids. It starts with us, caring about each other."

Central Du Page Health System

Central Du Page is located in Winfield, Illinois, near Chicago. Representing seven member organizations, it supports roughly 3,000 full-time and part-time employees. When Donald C. Sibery, president and CEO, took over its leadership two years ago, the system was very successful and stable; historically, it had experienced mostly incremental change. New challenges and future growth, however, required an ability to deal with rapid change. Sibery decided to facilitate the process by embarking on a cultural transformation process similar to one experienced at his former institution. The initial emphasis focused on senior management's leadership; current efforts are directed at implementing the process throughout the whole organization. This year's goal is to have 2,000 employees begin their own transformation journey.

Sibery reports definite organizational benefits in the two years since he joined Central Du Page. In the beginning, he recognized that he had very talented people on staff. His contribution was making new tools available to facilitate the great strides they wanted to make. The system's vision is for the communities they serve to be the healthiest in the United States by the year 2007. Accomplishing something of that magnitude is only possible if the staff meets two goals identified as crucial. First is to become a world-class listener (to stakeholders). And second is to become a world-class partner. They know that the first key to improved communication and better relationships is the ability to really listen to each other. This in turn will lead to the creation of new partnerships considered critical to their future success. Sibery knew from experience that going through a cultural transformation would help make the two goals a reality.

As with most health care delivery organizations, more than 80 percent of the workforce is female. Sibery and Barbara Lockwood, RN, vice president for patient care services, recognized the importance of understanding the differences in communication between males and females. Together, with the assistance of a consulting group, they designed Releasing the Feminine Spirit, a program specifically for female staff. Its purpose is to build a core group of women within the organization that will help to create a whole, healing, inclusive, and creative culture, enabling the group to serve the community beyond what was initially imagined. Sibery and Lockwood understand that women need to celebrate, grieve, and heal themselves first in order to better serve their patients. Lockwood believes that many women caregivers lack the support needed to keep them from functioning "on empty" much of the time. The program for female staff has been enormously successful and not only celebrates diversity but also builds community.

Sibery believes their work thus far has led to observable positive benefits in a number of areas. He believes that people are learning to hear one another and are developing an understanding of how others see the world. Senior management had to learn not to defend themselves but rather to take in others' feedback and opinions and to thank them for their comments. People are learning the difference between a dialogue and a discussion. Sibery views a discussion as a conversation in which people continue to hold on to their point of view without really listening to others. In a dialogue people are asked to suspend their own views to be open to other points of view. It is only in a dialogue that something new may occur. Most noticeable is the way people talk together about the future. Sibery considers most conversations to be probability discussions, which is to say that discussion is generally based on past experiences and as a result future possibilities aren't considered. Today, he says, this is reversed. He quotes an unknown author, "The past should be used as a guidepost and not a hitching post." Possibilities only reside in the future, and the future is where Central Du Page is spending most of its time.

Although the word *soul* has not been used in the organization, staff members do talk about heart and passion. Sibery believes that these words are interchangeable with soul. "Here, people are speaking from their heart and passion," says Sibery. "In a business world model, there is no room for emotion; our emotions are to be left at the front door or, better yet, at home. At Central Du Page, we are giving people permission to speak from their hearts. Out of that comes breakthrough performance."

Diane Boynton, director of human resources development, believes that if health care organizations want to develop and retain the best people, then they must create the working environment that fosters relatedness, authenticity, and wholeness in their lives. Everything has to be in support of that environment. "We bring our hearts to work" is their new theme—a reminder of the changing culture that has led to revamped employee recognition and performance programs. Employees and management are taking 100 percent responsibility for their growth and are obtaining feedback on their performance.

Relationships with the medical staff are very different today, Sibery reports. This change has enabled Central Du Page to put together a long-term managed care contract that accounts for 40 percent of its revenue stream. He emphasizes it would never have happened just a few years ago. The health system has also embraced physician leadership at the executive level. Today, five of the top twelve executive positions are filled by physicians, compared with one in the past. The number of medical directors is expanding, and the medical executive committee has reinvented itself. Although the committee continues to function in the traditional role of credentialing and risk management, it is also carrying the vision and mission of the system into the community.

Sibery admits they have lost some people in the process of cultural transformation. Some people didn't like the new culture and left, only to return after experiencing other facilities. Some have simply left. But, he adds, "The old culture used to drive people away also." Others, as a result of identifying their vocational passion, have realized that even though they have loved their time at Du Page, they are not doing their heart's desire. "We celebrate what they have done and support them in doing something else," says Sibery. "What better way to lose people?"

Beaver Dam Community Hospital
Selected as one of the 100 best hospitals in the United States in 1998, Beaver Dam Community Hospital is a small facility located in Beaver Dam, Wisconsin. John Landdeck, president, believes this honor is a direct outgrowth of the way hospital staff work together. Although the award criteria focus on clinical outcomes and risk management, he believes that employees are more alert and sensitive because of the hospital's internal culture, which he considers soulful.

"We use the word *soul* often," Landdeck says. He compares soul to the special feelings caregivers have when treating family and friends and believes the close feeling of personal relationship should be present in every interaction, whether treating a patient or talking with a salesperson. He suggests that every task can be addressed in a personal manner. Even cleaning floors takes on a different perspective if it is done as though a personal friend were going to come in the door.

The hospital embarked on its own soulful journey four or five years ago. Management believed that things were going well and that they were doing all the right things as an organization. However, an employee survey suggested something very different. Subsequently, management asked themselves three very important questions: "What is our management style? What is the culture? What should we be doing?" Follow-up work with outside consultants helped them to develop a culture in which caring for each other was central to everything being done.

The hospital encourages nurses to sit down and cry with a patient's family if it seems the right thing to do at the time. Landdeck cautions, "This is not to say that we do not carefully manage the facility. We do. We watch the number of FTEs and our productivity." But, he observes paradoxically, "The more time it takes to sit down with a patient, the more work gets done."

Landdeck believes the hospital's soulful culture significantly affects the relationships among all stakeholders, including patients, the community, employees, physicians, and the board. It has changed the organization's belief system about treating illness. In contrast with its previous approach, the hospital believes that it is not there merely to treat illness or injury nor just to seek perfect health. Rather, its task is to prepare people for the eventuality of death; the hospital helps people practice dying. The realization that each hospital and community member is mortal has led to a new belief system. Thus, it is fitting to care for people's needs not only in body but in mind, spirit, or whatever else is required. The nursing staff subsequently reorganized itself around this philosophy, with a new focus on the totality of an individual's health. An introductory alternative/complementary medicine program is a direct outgrowth of that focus, and the medical staff, for example, has become increasingly aware of the appropriateness of chiropractic medicine for some patients.

Landdeck is convinced that working together differently as a staff creates an organization in which people at all levels are aligned with its mission and success. Increased employee participation is obvious in everything from budgeting to capital expenditures. An employee group is responsible for assigning benefit dollars. Physicians are involved in deciding the hospital's direction as well as in purchasing, not just medical equipment and instrumentation, but laundry trucks too.

Distinct financial benefits are being reaped. Landdeck says that the hospital's financial performance is directly attributable to a number of projects spearheaded by various employee groups. One such example is the new sports medicine program designed by a multidisciplinary, voluntary employee group. Another group recommended combining two ultrasound units and thereby saving considerable money; staffing levels decreased while productivity and performance increased. Landdeck believes that measurable outcomes are attached to such projects. In addition, he believes that new projects exist because of the different way people behave and treat each other, which also makes a difference in how the hospital works with the community. The hospital is currently involved in a tobacco-free project and is working with educators, lawyers, businesses, and city government to promote an ordinance limiting the sale of tobacco products.

Landdeck also believes that the way the hospital and physicians work together is changing dramatically. For example, in the past the introduction of critical paths might have prompted physicians to become defensive; today, the physicians are not as prone to react negatively. The hospital's ability to partner with its physicians is also shifting; physicians now are more likely to initiate partnering opportunities. The orthopedists, for example, approached the hospital about developing a joint replacement program together. And astonishingly, some physicians have taken the initiative in discussing the formation of a physician-hospital organization. Their new relationship is doing much to counter the historically adversarial interaction usually found between hospitals and physicians.

Celebration Health, Florida Hospital System

Celebration Health in Orlando, part of the Florida Hospital System, began as a vision of health care for the twenty-first century. As CEO, Des Cummings recalls, "We started with a blank piece of paper. We wanted to take the best of what was in the Florida Hospital System and couple it with what could be." Its various services have opened over a period of months, beginning with The Fitness Center in November 1997 and followed by outpatient services, physician offices, imaging services, and the Women's Center in January 1998. The inpatient hospital wing, which became operational in July 1998, functions today as a learning laboratory for other hospitals.

Care of the whole person for the person's entire life best describes Celebration Health, says Cummings. The focus is on the whole person, not just on an episodic event. It is a philosophy that moves from a one-dimensional perspective—the illness or episode—to a three-dimensional one connecting the whole person—mind, body, and spirit. Cummings likened such a health care delivery model to an electric light. "The electricity is the spirit, the wiring the body, and the bulb, the mind. The light is the soul." He views soul as the synergy of the three dimensions. Soul is enhanced when the whole person is engaged.

Cummings believes that if hospitals are to be of value to society, health care for the future must be redefined. Cummings points out that today people may appreciate having the availability of a good hospital, but they hope that they don't have to use it because they only see the illness side. A redefined hospital can take on the role of helping people create a healthy lifestyle. Cummings believes that if we are to be able to solve people's health problems, we must educate them about lifestyle changes. To do this, hospitals must move from a crises-centered environment to one of a health center. The hospital becomes the holistic resource center that inspires people to health and where people want to go.

In support of its belief system, Celebration makes a considerable investment in staff education. Systems based on training and structure are emphasized to ensure sustainability. Every new employee is enrolled in Vitality Training, Celebration's training program based on the cornerstones of its mission— connecting mind, body, and spirit. Thereafter, one day each quarter is devoted to further training and team building, continually reenforcing each element. Employees develop their own strategies for implementing this training in their personal and work lives. They plan for

> *"Hospitals are the true melting pot, the common ground of the community where everyone comes for care at some point over the course of a lifetime. Everyone wants health. By creating health competencies, hospitals can become a destination and the soul of the community."*
>
> —Des Cummings, Jr., CEO, Business Development Division, Celebration Health
>
>

how they will influence the delivery of care. Physicians go through a similar process, determining how they will be responsible for Celebration's vision in the way they practice medicine.

Celebration Health developed a unique delivery model to meet its vision. Each of the hospital's inpatient rooms is licensed as a universal room; that is, each room can be qualified as an ICU, PCU, CCU, labor and delivery, and so on. This flexibility allows the hospital to redefine its beds according to need. Under the usual bed-use model, a patient who begins care in an ICU makes a step-down progression to a PCU and then to a medical surgical bed. In what Celebration describes as a machinelike model, rooms would have turned over three times with multiple staff changes. Celebration's approach provides a 10 to 15 percent increase in staffing productivity. The larger rooms allow more family support, and more relational nursing is possible because the staff doesn't change. In addition, the computerized charting done outside each room allows nurses more time to give patients full attention. The model's flexibility allows the hospital to be used more effectively.

Cummings admits that there is a large capital investment up front for the universal rooms, but they offer significant benefits to patients as well as financial savings to the hospital. As he says, capital expenditures are a one-time event; wages and operating expenses are an everyday event. Through its integrative services approach, the hospital achieves higher patient satisfaction and realizes a substantial cost savings.

The hospital's Women's Center is also based on a holistic, integrated model. With a lobby resembling a cross between a hotel and a Barnes & Noble reading area, it serves as both a resource and health center. There is an integrated delivery approach at every level, allowing every aspect of care, including diagnostic imaging, to be done in one place, which eliminates the necessity of patients dressing and undressing and registering more than once.

Every aspect of the hospital, including the lobby, is designed as a holistic environment speaking to the mind, body, and spirit. One atrium wall in the lobby features a nature video, offering a place of movement, peace, and renewal. Not to be forgotten, however, is the hospital's goal of making health fun and less intrusive, particularly for children. General Electric designed an MRI that allows a child to view a favorite video during the procedure. Because the child is relaxed and engaged in something fun, there is often no need for sedation and consequently the presence of a nurse. Thus, both staffing and medication cost savings are realized. But most important, with a less intrusive process the child is not fearful and has a better medical experience, which should be the goal in other areas too, Cummings believes.

CONCLUSION

*O*ur brief glimpse into these organizations reminds us what is possible. Their stories highlight the defining difference of organizations whose stakeholders work together in partnership. While honoring the past, each sees the future as something to be embraced. It takes considerable courage to fly in the face of business as usual and embrace a future of possibility. Though these organizations differ in size, location, and purpose, a crucial commonality characterizes their belief systems and the ways in which they operate. Acknowledging their passion and heart, recognizing the importance of relationship, creating an environment of respect and open communication—all nurture the organization's soul.

References

[1] Stephanie Gruner, "Have Fun, Make Money," *Inc.* (May 1998): 123.

[2] Kevin Freiberg and Jackie Freiberg, *Nuts!* (Auston, Tex.: Bard Press, 1996), p. 158.

[3] Brenda Palk Sunco, "How Fun Flies at Southwest Airlines," *Personnel Journal* 74, no. 6 (June 1995): 62.

[4] Freiberg and Freiberg, *Nuts!,* p. 158.

[5] Tom Chappell, *The Soul of a Business,* audiotape, conference on Rediscovering the Soul in Business, Boise, Idaho, September 1995.

[6] Tom Chappell, *The Soul of a Business* (New York: Bantam Books, 1993), pp. 32–33.

7   Ibid., pp. 148–49.

8   Ibid., p. 63.

9   "God and Toothpaste," *New York Times Magazine* (December 22, 1996): 26.

10 Irwin M. Rubin and Raymond Fernandez, *My Pulse Is Not What It Used to Be, The Leadership Challenges in Health Care* (Honolulu: Temenos Foundation, 1991), p. 7.

11 Richard Stone, *Nightime Stories* (Salt Lake City: Nightime Pediatrics Press, 1998), p. 42.

CHAPTER TEN

Developing Strategies for Reclaiming Soul

*"Throw caution to the wind and jump
into the midst of things today."*[1]
—Frederic and Mary Ann Brussat

$\mathcal{W}$e hope you now want to begin the journey yourself to find soul and to assist organizations in enhancing soulfulness. You might pose the same question as the woman who asked, "What can I do as one person to begin the journey?"

To suggest that one person can change an entire organization, or even solve some of the major problems, is to place an unrealistic burden on anyone. What we do suggest is that every person can affect her or his own life and can influence others. Believing otherwise precludes ever trying. In the following sections, we highlight a number of activities and strategies to guide you and offer suggestions for both individuals and organizations, though many are similar. Readers are free to create their own methodology; for those who feel a more formalized action plan would be helpful, we've provided an outline as a guide. The most important thing is to just begin!

CONFRONTING THE VOICE OF JUDGMENT

*A*llowing a belief to paralyze us only gives more power to the "Voice of Judgment (VOJ)," a phrase coined by Ray and Myers that describes the part of us that sabotages change and movement.[2] The

> *"Faced with the choice between changing one's mind and proving that there is no need to do so, almost everybody gets busy with the proof."*
>
> —John Kenneth Galbraith
>
>

VOJ judges, condemns, puts down, assigns guilt, and buries any action that deflects from the norm. So if the normal mode of operation is to be machine-like, to function as a cog in the wheel, and to operate in linear ways, any attempt to deviate will be attacked vigorously by that part of us that doesn't want to rock the boat. To put it another way, we seem to have a natural disposition to keep things the way we perceive our current reality to be.

We challenge you to reflect on how the VOJ conflicts with the soulful actions you may wish to initiate or influence in your organization. In figure 10-1, we invite you to add to some of the VOJ statements that paralyze us. Then rewrite the statement in a way that invites action. Such negative statements, when changed, empower a person to step out of the "box" and take a leap of faith.

FIGURE 10-1

Changing Perceptions Worksheet

Voice of Judgment	Change the Statement to:
• Management will never change.	
• The bottom line rules everything.	
• No one person can make a difference.	
• Don't rock the boat.	

TAKING THE LEAP

*N*othing makes us feel so alone as when we carry a burden or concern by ourselves. One of the key ingredients in being resilient in the face of adverse situations is our relationship with, and the support of, others. Within each organization can be found others with beliefs and frustrations similar to our own. We've talked with many people and conducted an informal focus group of health care professionals with diverse backgrounds. We were both surprised and delighted to find the intense interest in the topic of soul. Our discussion about soul and the qualities supporting it was meaningful and deep. As one focus group participant said, "We should do this every week." We agree! Such ongoing dialogue provides an opportunity to discuss issues not normally talked about in other professional settings. We suggest that before embarking on your journey to reclaim soul, find such a group, either within the organization or among other colleagues.

Then what actions can you take? The following process of strategy formulation will allow you to gather information vital to developing strategies and action plans to enhance soul in your career and/or organization.

IDENTIFYING POSITIVE AND NEGATIVE FORCES

*F*igure 10-2 offers a model for analyzing your current situation, moving forward toward a goal or sense of mission. It combines two analytical methodologies. The first is called force field analysis.[3] The second is a strategic planning tool known by the acronym SWOT (strengths, weaknesses, opportunities, threats).

The first step in this process, shown in the diagram, consists of having a clear understanding of your mission/goal. It involves developing a written description, or at least a mental picture, of what it means to be active in soulful work and/or in a soulful organization. (Chapter 9 contains examples of such organizations.)

FIGURE 10-2

Strategy Development

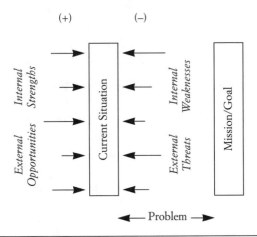

Copyright 1998 by James Henry.

There are ways of measuring some of the qualities of soul (individuality, career satisfaction, diversity, and community), such as through opinion surveys and the like.

The next step is to conduct a thorough analysis of your current situation. The gap between your current situation (what you have) and your mission/goal (what you want) is the definition of your problem. The bigger the gap between the two, the bigger the problem and the more energy and resources must be expended to achieve a positive result.

(+) Forces

Examining your current situation involves the identification of positive (+) forces and negative (–) forces influencing you. First, there are positive, driving forces that may propel you in the direction of your mission/goal. These forces represent strengths over which you have control. For an individual, they could be such strengths as education, on-the-job experience, and personal motivation. For an organization, they could be financial assets, an experienced workforce, or organizational history/tradition.

There are also external factors or opportunities beyond your control that are also driving forces. For an individual, these might be educational opportunities such as conferences, books, or Internet groups on spirit/soul in work. For an organization, these could be organizational development consultants or other business groups modeling soul, such as Tom's of Maine.

(–) Forces

Next, there are undoubtedly negative, restraining forces or weaknesses over which you have control but which prohibit movement toward a desired end result. For an individual they might be the lack of time or experience. For an organization, they could be limited financial resources or lack of commitment by certain departments.

Finally, there are external negative factors beyond your control, threats that may inhibit your progress. For an individual, they could be the indifference of top management or the threat of job loss. For an organization, they might be pressure from competition or insurance providers.

Intensity Level

Positive and negative forces can be of varying intensities. The intensity level of a particular force is indicated by the length of its arrow in figure 10-2. In any case, the challenge is to develop strategies that will help to

- enhance and take advantage of the positive forces influencing your situation, and
- eliminate or at least minimize the impact of negative forces.

Identifying Internal Strengths

Internal strategies represent positive forces over which you have control. Examples for the individual and the organization are shown below, along with strategies to capitalize on them.

Examples for an individual:

Strength	*Strategy*
Sarah has excellent organizational and facilitation skills.	She plans to seek out other interested employees and establish a discussion group on reclaiming soul in her organization.
John enjoys photography.	He offers to take photos at employee events for the bulletin board.

Examples for an organization:

Strength	*Strategy*
A few employees in the human resources department enjoy conducting research.	They collect information about appreciative inquiry and conduct a pilot project using AI techniques.
The organization has a rich and colorful history, with many interesting stories.	Collect some of the most eventful stories about the organization, put them in writing, and distribute them during new-employee orientation sessions.

Identifying External Opportunities

The second category of positive forces propelling you toward your mission/goal is external opportunities. These are factors over which you have no control but can take advantage of to enhance soul. You will probably need to conduct research to gather thorough information about external opportunities.

Examples for an individual:

Opportunity	Strategy
The organization offers a tuition reimbursement program.	Sarah will enroll in a certification program to become a career development specialist.
The group supports volunteer community service activities.	John decides to enhance his sense of community by joining others in a Habitat for Humanity project.

Examples for an organization:

Opportunity	Strategy
Although perhaps not using the word *soul,* more and more organizations are seeking a soul-enhanced health care environment.	The group will seek out and send representatives to conferences on enhancing soul in business.
In at least larger metropolitan areas, a number of educators are respected for their wisdom with respect to soul.	The hospital trustees will seek out a respected educator to serve along with them on the board.

Identifying Internal Weaknesses

All individuals and organizations have weaknesses. You control them in the sense that you could turn a weakness into a strength or you could develop strategies to compensate for them.

Examples for an individual:

Weakness	Strategy
Sarah is overloaded with debt as a result of obtaining education loans. She can't afford to move to a lower-paying but more soulful work environment.	Sarah will explore ways to simplify her lifestyle, cutting back on expenses and reducing her debt as quickly as possible.

Weakness
John has dedicated his entire life to his health care profession and has little sense of identity beyond his work.

Strategy
He commits himself to a self-exploration process, meeting weekly with a support group of his peers who are struggling with similar issues.

Examples for an organization:

Weakness
Extensive renovation would be required to create a more soulful physical atmosphere.

Strategy
Whenever possible, departments will encourage employees to personalize office space and decorate hallways in ways that reflect individuality and community.

Financial pressure makes it increasingly difficult to fund employee social events.

The organization will establish a spirit committee to solicit and implement ideas for social interaction within budgetary parameters.

Identifying External Threats
Finally, there are external threats to you or your work group over which you have no control but which might prevent you from achieving your goal of reclaiming soul. The task is to thoroughly identify and research these, then develop strategies to minimize their impact on you.

Examples for an individual:

Threat
Sarah recently received a mandate to spend no more than an average of 10 minutes per patient.

Strategy
Sarah will use her extensive research skills to identify alternative ways of providing health care services beyond a large institution.

Threat
John was informed there will be a 10 percent reduction in staff because of financial pressures and new technologies.

Strategy
John will seek out assistance and develop a plan for establishing his own business.

Examples for an organization:

Threat
There is an ongoing concern about a possible takeover or a merger with other health care organizations.

Strategy
Whenever possible, merger negotiations will include ways to take care of employees and preserve the soul of the organization.

There is a growing public demand for patient-friendly health care.

The organization will develop a strategic plan for maintaining and improving patient satisfaction in ways patients define as meaningful.

Developing Additional Strategies

As we have seen, strategies can be developed to build on the positive forces of strengths and external opportunities. Strategies may also be formulated to minimize the negative forces of weaknesses and external threats.

In the above examples, Sarah and John each developed four strategies to move toward their respective mission/goals and to enhance soul, and eight strategies were identified for the organization. However, there are virtually hundreds of possible strategies that could be formulated and implemented over a period of time. Time and cost factors will limit choices. On the other hand, reclaiming soul in health care does not necessarily need to be either costly or time-consuming. Often some seemingly casual and ordinary activities, practiced on a fairly regular basis, can heighten experience of soul. Especially for the individual, Moore's *The*

Reenchantment of Ordinary Life is packed with suggestions;[4] another resource is *100 Ways to Keep Your Soul Alive.*[5]

When facilitating planning sessions, Linda frequently asks members of the group to wave a magic wand and design the future as they would like to see it. Such a futuristic activity has the advantage of stepping out of the box of reality into one of possibility. We suggest that you, too, figuratively wave your wand over your organization. What do you want your particular organization to be? How do you want people to act? What would you like to see happen? Then work backward, retracing the steps it has taken to get there. Finally, where do you personally fit into the picture?

A MENU OF STRATEGIES

Listed below is a cafeteria menu of possible strategies for individuals and organizations. Many of them were mentioned earlier but are listed again to consolidate them in one place. They are organized according to the four qualities of soul and essentially represent strategies for individuals to implement, although organizations can do things to support the implementation. Suggestions on how to provide such organizational support are also offered.

Promoting Individuality

Complete the Myers-Briggs Type Indicator (MBTI®)   If you haven't already done so, this is an excellent place to begin learning more about yourself and connecting to soul. It can be accessed through the Internet, and a different version is included in the book *Please Understand Me II.*[6] Extremely well researched, the MBTI® provides feedback about your preferences for approaching both the internal and external world. For example, even though each of us can do both, Jim's preference is for introversion, seeking interconnectedness— and hence soul—through internal listening and processing ideas and experiences. On the other hand, Linda is more extraverted, making connections through interaction with the external world of people, things, and information. Neither preference is right or wrong. In fact, some data suggest that people are born with one preference or the other. Indeed, some strategies we suggest will appeal to you more than others depending on your MBTI® preferences.

For the Organization   The MBTI® could be included in training programs such as team building. Certification programs are offered throughout the year and in many different cities. Purchased in bulk, the Form G Self-Scorable version and the accompanying booklet, *Introduction to Type in Organizations,* can be purchased for about $10 a person.[7]

Engage in Lifelong Learning   Because of advances in technology and the information explosion, career success mandates continuing growth and education in technical areas. However, it's equally important to increase one's knowledge and skills in the softer disciplines such as leadership and human relations. Today, many organizations are giving equal weight to these skills in contrast with technical abilities.

For the Organization   Establish a tuition reimbursement program covering the softer disciplines as well as technical areas. Again, many excellent courses are offered at community colleges at reasonable expense.

Examine Your Belief System   Your beliefs are easy to identify simply by reflecting on admonitions, "shoulds," and "oughts" communicated in one form or another by significant adults when you were a child. Even if not difficult to identify, these messages usually contain weighty energy so that attempting to act in opposition to them often results in reexperiencing fear and anxiety.

One of Jim's messages, for example, was "Work hard, be responsible, and you'll get ahead." The power of this assumption influenced his behavior and goals for many years until he was able to let go and at times enjoy simply "being."

Linda's message was simple: "Be good." Without breaking the law or harming herself or others, releasing some of the energy of this message involved going against certain parental norms.

Share Your Personal Story Whenever Possible and Appropriate
Your story shared and listened to without judgment can result in a profoundly soulful adventure. Of course, some of one's life experiences are so private that they are to be shared only in an intimate relationship, but you have control over what is revealed. Often, one story sparks the recollection of similar events among your audience, helping people to connect soulfully with one another.

For the Organization   An organization can promote story telling in a number of ways. Stories can be included regularly in newsletters and on bulletin boards, and can be shared through e-mail. As mentioned earlier, Tom's of Maine sets aside special times when employees share life events and stories about themselves.

Stories about the past as well as the present are invaluable. The story of the Southwest Airlines' flight attendant who hid in a luggage bin, offering a drink to a surprised passenger, is worthy of repeated sharing. Specific employees, such as those in the training department, could be enlisted to share organizational stories.

Still another way to preserve the past is through the publication of a history of the institution, which could be given out during new-employee orientation.

Disassociate Yourself from Your Identity   An opposite strategy to the preceding one is detaching yourself from your story or identity. It is the negation of a self-image, role, or particular status enjoyed in the community, which can be a very frightening experience but can lead to a deeper sense of who you are.

Many health care professionals, for example, invest years of hard work and expense to achieve licensing or certification. A significant part of their identity hinges on their profession, so its loss may be very disorienting. This is why, long after retirement, Mr. Smith continues to insist on being called doctor. Or why, long after we become adults, most of us would choke at the thought of calling our parents by their first names.

As a strategy, consider taking a vacation or sabbatical from your professional role. By yourself, visit a place or involve yourself in a community where no one knows who you are. Don't reveal your profession; simply say, "I'm on vacation and would rather not talk about what I do for a living." If you do this, it's probably wise to have a coach or support system available afterwards for a debriefing of the experience and the feelings associated with it.

Using an Active Imagination, Change Your Name   This is a severe step and certainly would bewilder your family and friends. Nonetheless, identify your most admired hero or heroine, someone not associated with your current profession, and examine whether this deeply admired person represents your shadow. Make a list of the specific characteristics you associate with this person. Stand outside of yourself, so to speak, and ask which of these characteristics could possibly be an expression of yourself. Another, related activity seeks input of close friends and relatives: ask them to select a celebrity with characteristics similar to some of yours.

Keep a Journal   A journal is an ongoing narrative of both your inner and outer life experiences; in fact, a whole technology is associated with this strategy. Ira Prokoff in particular pioneered "journaling," and there are people licensed to teach various techniques.

The beauty is that you can share your most private thoughts and feelings with yourself without fear of exposure.

If, along with others, Carl Jung is correct in the perception that we all have an inner self possessing great wisdom, then we can be our own therapists. You can even personalize the self and give it a name of your liking. In his journal, Jim especially enjoys the technique of dialogue, which he carries on with the imaginary Chris, and it goes something like this:

> *Jim:* "I'd like to talk to you about the book I'm writing with Linda."
> *Chris:* "It's about time. I've been waiting to discuss it with you. Are you having a problem?"
> *Jim:* "Yes, I'm scared that no one will want to read it."
> *Chris:* "Well, as you know, I'm looking over your shoulder as you write. I'm quite impressed."

And so on. Some may view this as a rather weird strategy. Indeed, it must be used in conjunction with other methods of getting feedback, especially when writing a book. But if another inner voice were in charge, such as the Voice of Judgment, neither of us would even attempt this project.

Try Meditation   Many meditative methods are available for your consideration. You might concentrate on a relatively neutral object such as a candle. You could engage in a guided meditation, either alone or with the help of a facilitator. Or you could use a mantra of some kind, such as a rosary or knitting.

A notable amount of evidence exists today showing that meditation affects our brain waves. Through the use of some feedback mechanisms, such as EEG biofeedback, meditation is being used to treat several dysfunctions, such as attention deficit disorder. We also know it can affect the physiology of the body—lowering blood pressure, for example.

Work with Your Dreams   It is quite helpful to do this in conjunction with a professional, such as a Jungian analyst, but even without professional guidance, you may grow in self-understanding through this strategy.

Everyone dreams. The dreams can be explored by disciplining oneself to write them down on paper. Simply keep a notebook by the bed and record the dream immediately on awakening.

Every element in a dream represents a part of one's personality. The following is an example:

> I am sitting at my desk when suddenly a doctor comes storming through the door. He is furious because I failed to complete some paperwork on a patient of his. He tells me to report immediately to the hospital administrator. Next, I enter the administrator's office. Cold and without emotion, he glares at me with his steely eyes. He says that one more mistake like this and I'm fired. As I leave his office, his secretary gazes upon me empathetically. "Don't worry," she says. "He is really a pussycat underneath that icy exterior and couldn't fire anyone if he had to."

All parts of this dream reveal aspects of this individual's vast unknown. Characteristics of the furious doctor, the icy administrator, and the empathetic secretary surface from the unconscious and could be part of the dreamer's makeup. Accepting and embracing the characteristics enhance the dreamer's sense of individuality and soul.

For the Organization   Low-cost brown-bag programs on journal writing, meditation, and dreams could be provided for employees to attend on a voluntary basis. Many organizations offer physical wellness events, so why not soul wellness? The more employees individuate and become conscious of themselves, the more their creative energy is released. On the other hand, people who follow a herd instinct, especially when the herd hardens itself against the corporation's health and mission, can inflict significant damage.

Kill the Voice of Judgment   Earlier we suggested that every truth has a contrasting opposite. The opposite of individuality is totalitarianism and its voice is the VOJ. It seeks to terrorize you and keep you bound to herd mentality. It oppresses growth and creativity. Whether originating in you or in others, it seeks to administer critical blows to your intrinsic self-worth. It anesthetizes soul.

Therefore, you must attack the VOJ and kill it. When you hear the VOJ in yourself, write a nasty letter to it. Then, crumple the letter and throw it in the trash. Make it look ridiculous and laugh at it. Remember times when you went against the VOJ or the norm of the day and were successful in the face of it.

Comedian Ronnie Shakes once said, "I was going to buy a copy of *The Power of Positive Thinking,* and then I thought: What the hell good would that do?" That, dear reader, is the VOJ attempting to keep us in bondage.

Advancing Career Satisfaction

Explore and Assess a New Career   The amount of time this takes depends on several factors. How much are you enjoying your career and job? What do you anticipate the future to be in your field? Is your particular work environment changing and increasing your dissatisfaction? (We suggested earlier that health care is changing dramatically.)

Career assessment can take anywhere from a few hours, perhaps by enrolling in a community college program, to a year-long search for vocational direction. If additional education is required, the transition to a new vocation may take several years. Much depends on a person's motivation, available time, and financial resources. In any case, many career programs and resources are available to assist you, especially in urban areas (refer to chapter 6).

For the Organization   Offering career exploration and development programs is an excellent means of assisting employees to find the satisfaction in their career that can lead to greater productivity. In addition, in terms of human resources and job placement, perhaps nothing is more expensive than putting a square peg in a round hole. Offering career development services need not be time-consuming and expensive; at the very least, most community colleges offer these services.

Do Nothing!   Yes, this really is a strategy. Procrastination is not necessarily a bad thing. Sometimes an inner voice urges us: "Don't just do something; stand there." This could be a time for letting go and letting things happen. Reflecting over time, one may conclude, "Yes, this is the direction I must go." Or you may wish to explore a few options before committing to a course of action.

Go into Business for Yourself   Some people, like management guru Peter Drucker, are now predicting that in 10 or 20 years the largest business organization will have no more than 200 permanent employees. Everyone else will be contract temporary workers. Even today, the largest for-profit corporation is Manpower, which specializes in placing temporary employees, and roughly 40 percent of Microsoft workers are contracting their services.

Given these trends, it behooves us to begin working on a career plan for "You Inc." Even if you're currently employed, now is the time to shift your perspective and view your employer as your customer. You receive payment for services rendered, and when these services are no longer needed, you take your business elsewhere. You Inc. "implies being self-accountable, self-directed, self-responsible, self-motivated and having the attitude of being self-employed whether inside or outside a health care organization."[8]

Take Moderate Risks   Risk analysis is a helpful planning tool that can be used as a reality check. It serves as a way to subjectively estimate the degree of hazard involved in achieving a goal. Estimating risk is especially helpful in the midst of a changing health care environment.

We define moderate risk in the following manner. Suppose you have a 95 percent chance of success in making a career change and only a 5 percent chance of failure. Your goal is achievable with hardly any effort. On the other hand, what if you have only a 5 percent chance of success? You undoubtedly are setting yourself up for failure. Moderate risk is defined as taking 50–50 chances. With at least a 50 percent chance of success in achieving a goal, your effort may be worth making. Of course, the level of risk associated with a possible course of action is a subjective estimate, but remember nonetheless that the higher the risk, the more likely you will end up being disappointed.

Join a Support Group When Planning a Career Exploration and Transition   As part of her doctoral program, Mary Lynn Pulley interviewed dozens of people who had successfully moved from losing their job to new employment or a new career. She reports three essential factors contributing to their success.[9] All of them (1) have an active faith system of one kind or another, (2) possess resiliency, the ability to accept change and bounce back from loss, and (3) belong to a highly supportive community. This support community may consist of friends and family or perhaps it's a group of people themselves going through a career change and providing encouragement for one another.

Activate Your Faith   According to polls, more than 90 percent of the population believe in some form of universal being. By faith we don't refer to belief in a particular doctrine or theology only but to that which motivates action—a trust that we are being led by "hidden hands."

In a dialogue in a TV series between Bill Moyers and Joseph Campbell on *The Power of Myth*, which was subsequently published in a book, Moyers asked, "[Are we] being helped by hidden hands?" Campbell replied, "All the time . . . if you follow your bliss you put yourself on a kind of track that has been there all the while, waiting for you, and the life you ought to be living is the one you are living."[10]

Prayer is a particular form of activating one's faith. In his many books, Larry Dossey, MD, offers convincing testimony that prayer makes a difference. It is not recommended for merely getting God's attention or pulling God's string. Use your own metaphor for the divine, but we recommend an approach something like this: "God, as you know, I am really struggling with my sense of vocational direction. I would really like your guidance, and I am promising in advance to pay attention." Of course, the key task is to pay attention to the events of the following days and weeks.

Simplify Your Life   During workshops and other presentations, we are sometimes confronted with statements similar to this one: "That's all well and good. But how do you follow your bliss when you are a single parent with two kids? I don't particularly like my job, but someone must put food on the table." Our response, first of all, is to indicate a preference for the word *passion* instead of the word *bliss* because bliss implies that following one's vocational calling is not hard work. Second, raising two kids to become healthy adults is at least part of one's calling that can be joyful as well as challenging. Finally, one can take steps today, such as pursuing additional education, that can lead to a deeper experience of vocational calling in the future when the children are grown.

Contrary to the old PaineWebber commercial (we are paraphrasing it), the quality of life (and one's connectedness to soul) is not necessarily dependent on the quality of one's investments and possessions. Except for the basic necessities of food, clothing, and shelter, the less we possess, the more freedom we enjoy.

For many people, living simply means simply living. Books abound on the why and the how of living a life of simple abundance less cluttered with things. Experiencing soul is not an expensive pursuit.

Honoring Diversity

Increase Your Compassion for Nature   Nature is alive with soul. When nature degenerates under the weight of civilization, soul diminishes as well. The word *compassion* literally means "to suffer with." Compassion begins with a deepening recognition of inter-connectedness. Nature is our neighbor, who needs to be treated in a neighborly way. When we do, nature shares her soul with us and gives us her bounty.

For those just beginning the pilgrimage of deepening apprecia-tion for nature, an excellent place to begin is Wilson's Pulitzer Prize-winning book *The Diversity of Life,* which stimulates wonder as it describes the incredible variety of the living world and how it came to be this way.[11]

Go on a Nature Retreat   After reading some books or perhaps exploring the diversity of nature through the Internet, do some field work. Go on a retreat into nature, preferably traveling to some exotic place where you have never been before. Examine carefully the diversity of the soil, rocks, vegetation, and moving creatures. All lessons about the soul begin here because the rhythms of nature began long before we humans appeared on earth.

We have said that mystery characterizes the essence of soul, and any sensitive health care provider instinctively knows this. The more deeply we explore nature, the more mysterious it becomes.

Therefore, a retreat into nature is like living a mystery novel instead of reading it.

Plant a Garden   Moore defines a garden "as the meeting of raw nature and the human imagination in which both seek the fulfillment of their beauty."[12] As we were writing these words, it was summer, a marvelous time of the year in the Northwest. We often write in the backyard, pausing to enjoy our garden. We witness the majestic evergreen trees touching the cloudless sky. We smell the roses and the sugary fragrance of the sweet peas climbing a trellis. In the early evening we pick snap beans, squash, carrots, and tomatoes for our dinner. Even our occasional dinner guests comment on how remarkably different freshly picked vegetables taste.

Each morning Jim begins the day with coffee in the garden, examining the garden closely to see which new flowers have emerged. It is a time of peace, a time when time itself seems to slow its pace.

You can begin your garden without having to worry about the depth of your knowledge or experience. Begin, as you may have as a child, with quickly maturing radishes. Plant the easy-to-grow flowers first: marigolds, California poppies, cosmos, daffodils, and gladiolas. You will quickly learn how responsive nature is to your care.

Bring Nature to Your Workplace   Many offices, filled with standard chairs, a desk, and bookcases, lack even a modicum of diversity. Many are colored in businesslike beige with uniformity of tone and hue. So if you can, diversify. Bring plants and flowers to your work location. Individualize your office with pictures and mementos reflecting your personal passion and experiences.

We have heard of a woman who, shortly after beginning a new job, came to the office one Sunday and painted her walls to her liking. Of course, people were astounded on Monday, but she simply explained that if there was a policy against such redecoration, she was unaware of it.

For the Organization   Encourage employees to bring nature into the workplace. Rather than enlisting the services of expensive decorators, why not ask for volunteers to serve on a nature-in-work project after establishing financial parameters. Because gardening has become a popular national pastime, many employees could bring offerings from their backyards.

Diversify Your Friendships   Make conscious efforts to broaden your circle of acquaintances. Variety is indeed the spice of life. Because many of us spend so much of our waking hours at work, the workplace provides an excellent opportunity for seeking diversity in relationships, which now is even easier as organizations actively pursue employee diversity.

Many of us make elaborate plans to spend vacations in foreign countries, not aware that to some degree exposure to other cultures may be only a few steps away in the office. Jim has been especially blessed with cross-cultural exposure through providing career planning services to a broad range of employees. For example, when a 68-year-old man born in Vietnam was informed that his job as an auditor was being eliminated, he stated during a visit with Jim, "I want to work another 20 years, but I wish to do something different." The last we heard, he was going to start his own business as a cross-cultural communications consultant.

For the Organization   Whenever possible, make conscious efforts to ensure that work and project teams reflect diversity because, apart from government regulations, it makes enormous business sense.

Fostering Community
Many of the strategies listed above will also foster community. Diversifying your acquaintances, for example, will serve to build

community. A few additional ways to enhance soul through expanding friendships and community are listed below.

Celebrate Together   Use every opportunity to celebrate special times as well as more mundane events. Encourage different members of your group or department to plan and take responsibility for such events.

For the Organization   Reconsider funding allocations for picnics, Christmas parties, and the like. Larger organizations often spend hundreds of thousands of dollars on these functions, but they are so large that little in the way of community is nurtured through them. Resources might be better used by establishing a spirit or soul committee and providing it with a budget. Identifying creative ways to foster community among workers and their families is a valid committee role. We suspect that such an approach will be quite cost-effective.

Increase Your Knowledge and Use of Communication Skills   Developing a sense of community is difficult if people fail to practice listening, paraphrasing, problem-solving, negotiation, and conflict resolution skills. Using such skills must be continually reinforced during meetings because it's easy for people to revert to ineffective communication habits.

Developing a Structured Action Plan
The information provided in this chapter is a concrete guide for developing a specific action plan. We recommend you use a notebook to record action strategies. And even though there's no right or wrong way of getting started, we suggest that the following steps can be used as a road map. Remember, road maps are of value simply as a way of getting from point A to point B and are not written in stone. Rather, they should be flexible enough to change if the road suddenly is under construction!

Step 1—My Support Group   In your notebook, list the individuals you consider important members of your support group. These are the people with whom you share mutual respect and trust. You know they will support you and your ideas.

Step 2—My Magic Wand   Write a scenario or vision of what a soulful group would look like in the future. Complete the following sentences:

I want my organization to be . . .

People will act . . .

The most important characteristics of our relationship will be . . .

In other words, describe in detail what this world will look like. There are no boundaries to envisioning.

Step 3—Kill the Voice of Judgment   Using figure 10-1, complete and expand this exercise. After listing as many VOJs as apply in your particular circumstance, change each of the statements to a positive one.

Step 4—Identify Your Personal Goal   Clearly identify your own personal goal or mission in this process.

Step 5—My Sphere of Influence   Fill in the columns suggested below, listing those individuals with whom you have some degree of influence, including people you supervise, peers, supervisors, clients, and so on. Then note the degree to which you have influence. For example, you may have a high degree of influence with those you supervise but, on the other hand, only a moderate level of influence with your peers. Finally, select the strategy you plan to employ in building an awareness of soul with each person.

Name   Relationship   Degree of Influence   Strategy to Make a Difference

Step 6—SWOT Using the model presented earlier in this chapter, identify the strengths, weaknesses, opportunities, and threats in your situation. Then, from the cafeteria menu of suggested strategies, select those that you plan to use for each of the areas identified above. You may find other strategies you wish to employ.

Step 7—Action Steps Select 10 or more action strategies that you personally can implement. Then list them in the columns below in the order of their importance. As an example, figure 10-3 shows eight strategies listed according to their priority.

Finally, write your plan of action. You may wish to assign a time line for each strategy so that you can check your progress. It will look something like this:

I will

enhance my own soul by . . .

enhance soul in my staff by . . .

enhance soul with my peers by . . .

encourage soul with my supervisory management by . . .

FIGURE 10-3

Action Steps

Most Important

Seek out other interested employees and establish a discussion group in the organization.

Explore ways to simplify my lifestyle, cutting back on expenses and reducing debt as quickly as possible.

Expand my circle of friendships by participating in a Habitat for Humanity project.

Seek out sources of information and develop a plan for establishing a personal business.

Least Important

Enroll in a certification program to become a career development specialist.

Identify alternative ways of providing health care services beyond large organizations.

Decorate the office space with photos that are especially soulful.

Complete a course on journal writing and write in a journal at least twice a week.

> *"We are not in control of
> life, and no matter how
> hard we try, the caprices of
> nature will win out over
> man. We can never predict
> what the outcome of an
> encounter will be. We can,
> however, exercise some
> control by participating in
> the process of our lives."*[13]
>
> —Arnold R. Beisser

CONCLUSION

$\mathcal{W}$e have suggested numerous activities to guide you in creating your action plan. As you proceed, you may find other strategies. Above all, your action plan is a means for reclaiming or enhancing soul in your life and/ or in health care. Perhaps it will represent the point of departure for a new journey. It may serve as a personal or organizational guide, unbounded by past perceptions and assumptions.

References

[1] Frederic Brussat and Mary Ann Brussat, *100 Ways to Keep Your Soul Alive, Living Deeply and Fully Every Day* (San Francisco: HarperSanFrancisco, 1994), p. 63.

[2] Michael Ray and Rochele Myers, *Creativity in Business* (New York: Doubleday, 1986).

[3] Kurt Lewin, *Resolving Social Conflicts, Field Theory in Social Science* (Washington, D.C.: American Psychological Association, 1997).

[4] Thomas Moore, *The Reenchantment of Ordinary Life* (New York: HarperCollins, 1996).

[5] Brussat and Brussat, *100 Ways.*

[6] David Keirsey, *Please Understand Me II* (Del Mar, Calif.: Prometheus Nemesis Books, 1998).

[7] Sandra Krebs Hirsh and Jean M. Kummerow, *Introduction to Type in Organizations* (Palo Alto, Calif.: Consulting Psychologist Press, 1990).

8 Todd Pearson, "Physician Employees: The 'New Social Contract' in Healthcare," *Career Planning and Adult Development Journal* 14, no. 1 (spring 1998): 48.

9 Mary Lynn Pulley, *Losing Your Job—Reclaiming Your Soul* (San Francisco: Jossey-Bass, 1997).

10 Joseph Campbell with Bill Moyers, *The Power of Myth* (New York: Doubleday, 1988).

11 Edward O. Wilson, *The Diversity of Life* (Cambridge, Mass.: The Belknap Press of Harvard University Press, 1992).

12 Thomas Moore, *Care of the Soul* (New York: HarperCollins, 1992), p. 96.

13 Arnold R. Beisser, *A Graceful Passage* (Des Plaines, Ill.: Bantam Doubleday, 1990).

Epilogue

Each lifetime is the pieces of a jigsaw puzzle.
For some there are more pieces.
For others the puzzle is more difficult to assemble.

Some seem to be born with a nearly completed puzzle.
And so it goes.
Souls going this way and that.
Trying to assemble the myriad parts.

But know this. No one has within themselves
All the pieces of their puzzle.
Like before the days when they used to seal
jigsaw puzzles in cellophane. Insuring that
All the pieces were there.

Everyone carries with them at least one and probably
Many pieces to someone else's puzzle.
Sometimes they know it.
Sometimes they don't.

And when you present your piece
Which is worthless to you,
To another, whether you know it or not,
Whether they know it or not,
You are a messenger from the Most High.

Excerpt from *Honey from the Rock: An Easy Introduction to Jewish Mysticism* by Lawrence Kushner (Woodstock, Vt.: Jewish Lights Publishing, 1990). Permission granted by Jewish Lights Publishing, P.O. Box 237, Woodstock, Vt. 05091, telephone 800-962-4544.

*H*ow better to conclude this brief journey together than to end with this moving poem? This is but another way of emphasizing interconnectedness. Throughout *Reclaiming Soul in Health Care,* we have offered a mere glimpse into the possibilities of reclaiming the heart and passion of our chosen work. We began with an exploration of soul, suggesting that it is a mysterious, magnificently unbounded, living web. Or, if you will, we could see soul as a living, three-dimensional jigsaw puzzle composed of thousands of interconnected pieces.

Having identified characteristics that personify the soulful organization, we described some of the major qualities of soul as they can be reclaimed and enhanced in health care. Each of these qualities contributes to the others, forming a photograph of what health care might look like in the helping professions. Later, we shared the stories of organizations that are concrete examples of people working together soulfully. They demonstrate that soul is not simply an abstract concept limited to theoretical textbooks. These organizations are alive and dancing before us, giving us hope for the future of health care. Soulful organizations can survive and flourish even in today's ever-changing and competitive environment.

Finally, we have suggested ways in which individuals and organizations can develop an intentionality—a purposefulness—about making a difference. Chapter 10 offered a menu of strategies to enhance soul, individually and in institutions. From our dialogues with others, we know that you'll discover other creative and meaningful strategies. We also recognize that the action plan offered here is a beginning only of what we know will be a very soulful journey. We encourage you to communicate with us, sharing your stories of how soul is being enhanced personally and in your organization. We can be reached on the Internet at jlhenry@aol.com.

Now, we invite you to begin.

Appendix

Team Building in a Health Care Setting

$\mathcal{A}$s noted in chapter 10, the Myers-Briggs Type Indicator (MBTI®) is an excellent tool for enhancing the qualities of soul in an organization. We used it as part of a team-building session in a 43-bed hospital in a medium-sized community. Nine members of key management and the board of directors participated, all of them completing the MBTI® before the meeting and forwarding their respective profiles to us.

Figure A-1 illustrates the type of feedback the group received. Names have been changed to maintain confidentiality. First, feedback is constructed around the four functions. They are offered as two sets of opposites in a quadrated circle, again a symbol of wholeness or completeness.

The two functions shown on the vertical axis represent different ways of receiving information. Everyone has access to all of these functions, but most people have preferences. Some people prefer to use their senses when receiving information, their sight, hearing, touch, and so on. To use a common metaphor, they tend to focus on the trees and not the forest. They tend to be practical, down-to-earth, and oriented to the way things are in their receptivity to information. They pay attention to facts, what's happening at the moment, and step-by-step processes.

FIGURE A-1

Hospital Board and Key Managers: Myers-Briggs Preferences

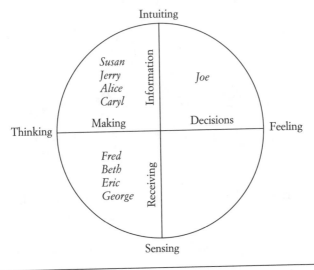

Other people prefer the function opposite to sensing, which is intuition, a kind of sixth sense. Referring again to the metaphor, they focus on the forest and not the trees. They enjoy searching for patterns in the information they are receiving, paying attention to the way things *could* be. They have valuable insights and like to search for future possibilities, making novel leaps in applying information in new and sometimes unusual ways.

On the horizontal axis, two contrasting ways of making decisions are shown. People with a thinking orientation make decisions based on hard data, statistics, financial analysis, and the like. They use rather impersonal reasoning and tend to be firm-minded.

On the other hand, those with a preference for feeling make decisions based on how those decisions affect others. Feeling doesn't mean emotional. The feeling function is really a valuing function.

These people enjoy relating to and working with others. They are sociable and friendly and are often able to detect the various moods and emotions of others and make decisions accordingly.

Those familiar with the MBTI® know that some people also prefer receiving information (called perceiving functions), while others prefer to make decisions (judging functions). In addition, imagine there is a third axis through the center of the quadrated circle in a perpendicular or upright fashion. This would be the extravert/introvert axis, meaning some people get their energy by focusing on the external world. Others become energized by getting "into their heads" and dealing with experiences, emotions, and information internally.

For ease in explaining, we take a shortcut and work with only the functions in four quadrants: NT (intuitive/thinking), NF (intuitive/feeling), SF (sensing/feeling), and ST (sensing/thinking). What follows is a brief description of the characteristics and strengths of people in a work setting according to their quadrant:

- *NTs.* People in this group are known for their competency and knowledge. They particularly enjoy ideas and concepts. They focus on the future, analyzing possibilities in an almost impersonal way. They are talented in developing strategies and linking various business and/or technological systems. They enjoy debating issues with an impeccable logic. In organizations, they often show up in strategic types of jobs, such as business analysis, research and development, or information systems. In health care, they may surface as psychiatrists, neurologists, cardiologists, biomedical researchers, or strategic managers.
- *NFs.* People in this quadrant tend to seek meaning and authenticity in work. They are superb at promoting harmony in work groups, especially if their innovative spirit is supported. They communicate with appreciation and enthusiasm. They provide insight into people issues and are especially adept at working with diverse

groups. They especially enjoy having fun during work and can make group educational events more interesting. In organizations, they often gravitate into marketing, public relations, human resources (employee relations), and training. In health care, they may be found in alternative medicine as nutritionists, speech pathologists, mental health counselors, or massage therapists.

- *SFs.* These people enjoy helping people in practical ways with everyday concerns. They are good at step-by-step processes that have valuable outcomes for others. They excel at applying experience to the job and in reviewing plans with others. They tend to be dependable and realistic in their approach to work. In organizations, they can be found in customer service, recruiting, education, and administrative positions. In health care, they tend to be nurses, medical/dental assistants, medical records administrators, receptionists, or primary care physicians.

- *STs.* These people find themselves drawn to work in which they can apply facts and experience. They excel at cause-and-effect thinking. They enjoy using proven methods and monitoring progress with data. They bring efficiency and quality-control skills to the job. In organizations, they can be found in operational positions as supervisors and in accounting, purchasing, and manufacturing. In health care, they appear as EEG technologists, emergency medical technicians, surgeons, administrators, and pharmacists.

BOARD AND MANAGER PROFILES

Returning to figure A-1, note that eight of the nine members of the board and senior management team are either NTs or STs, which is not uncommon. In a compilation of data involving more than 5,000 senior managers, 93 percent of them had a preference for the thinking function.[1] The one member of the team who preferred making decisions with the feeling function was a board member. Consider this reality in light of the makeup of the hospital's workforce: some 80 percent of the employees are female, and 60 percent of women prefer the feeling function. This percentage is undoubtedly even higher in health care. SFs in particular tend to gravitate to such jobs in health care as nursing.

A second point of interest is that more than 80 percent of the people who generally make health care decisions are female. In light of these facts, the management team found that the composite MBTI information shed light on how the hospital will conduct business.

Focusing attention only on the thinking function, the information in table A-1 summarizes how business is generally conducted by these hospital leaders. The center column reveals what may

TABLE A-1

Ways to Counteract Overextended Strengths

Strengths	Strengths Overextended	Actions That May Be Needed
Making decisions based on logic and impersonal analysis	"Damn the torpedoes. Full steam ahead." "I decide—you perform."	Seek consensus when appropriate and when buy-in is critical.
Setting goals objectively by determining what is to be achieved and how it will impact the bottom line	Focusing entirely on results and overlooking long-term implications; unyielding	Determine subjectively whom the goal will affect and how it will be received.
Solving problems by weighing the pros and cons of alternatives	A know-it-all expert blind to alternative solutions	Consider points of agreement first; seek many alternatives.
Communicating by being concise, using impersonal reasoning	Overly critical and picky with details; aloof	Share emotions as appropriate (not just anger); seek involvement and a variety of opinions.
Solving conflict by seeking objective clarity	Controlling and unyielding; "My way or the highway"	Solve conflicts by considering their impact on group harmony.

happen when the board and the managers find themselves pressured and under stress. Items in this column are shown as strengths overextended, which could be considered weaknesses. The right-hand column lists actions that could be taken to counteract weaknesses and adopt a more feeling approach to conducting business. Such actions are especially critical considering the makeup of the workforce and the female decision-making public.

RECLAIMING SOUL: TARA BRUIN'S STORY

$\mathcal{T}$ara Bruin (her pen name) was born with an inner passion for music and poetry already complete in her "acorn." "It's as though if I didn't write it down I would lose my mind." Her story includes the doctor in the delivery room examining her long, slender fingers and declaring that she would be a pianist. At age 4, the same doctor listened as Tara played a toy piano and excitedly declared that she had a perfect pitch.

By age 9, her inner harmony found expression in the form of poems. "I saw poetry as songs . . . which explains why some of my poetry is written like verses and then a chorus which is repeated at times."

Jim first met Tara as a teller in a tiny financial center located in a store in Scappoose, Oregon, northwest of Portland along the Columbia River. "I married at 19 and had four children by 23. I had to work, so even though I hated it, office/customer service/cash handling became my so-called career."

Vocational assessment indicated Tara's strong social and artistic interests. When Jim asked to see a sample of her poetry, she produced a one-and-a-half-inch binder filled with poems. Her MBTI® profile revealed Tara's slightly intraverted, highly intuitive, and feeling strengths.

The years 1997 and 1998 were pivotal—that's when Tara committed herself to reclaiming her soul. She mustered the courage to submit two poems in contests, and both were published. *Beyond* was published in the Amherst Society's annual anthology and *Just Love* made it into an annual anthology published by the American Poetry Guild.

During this period, Tara became quite active in the community. She led a grass-roots group to begin an affiliation with Habitat for Humanity. She joined the local Community Action Team's board of directors, then was appointed to the Northwestern Oregon Housing Authority Board.

Tara's transition has not come without emotional pain. She quit her job at the bank. The turmoil of change resulted in a separation from her husband. However, she commented, "Leading a life away from your soul's calling, away from the inner light of creativity, leads to self-destruction. . . . For my family and myself, I choose to follow the call as best as I am able." She has completed *Sensitive to Life,* her collection of poems, and hopes to get it published.

Tara's story is unique, as is everyone's. We could share dozens of other fascinating stories of people seeking to connect with soul and the soul's calling. Essentially, we chose Tara's story because of her poem, shared below, about the wolf, a Northwest Native American's metaphor for the inner self.

To Run with the Wolf

The wind pushes back my hair
Peals the frown from my face
The sunbeams meet with my body
My skin revels in it's warmth
My heart beats joyously

Clouds fly past, hurried
Chasing each other across the sky
Trees blur by on either side
As if my feet never touch ground
My hand reaches next to me
And I find him there, faithfully.

To be his friend
The highest honor
To protect
And be protected
We play and tease
Like family
Yet, I hoped
To run with the wolf.

I have known him since youth
Have learned so much from his maturing
People think the wolf wild, heathen
They are so very wrong
He is civilized, socialized
Wastes nothing, not even life.

I hear the soulful call
His voice beckoning
I feel the pull to follow
My spirit aches to fly
I reach instinctively
Freedom finding me.

He accepts me, a member of his pack
Our families joined in spirit
I can't imagine world without wolf
All of earth so dependent
Lose one, we all will follow
Eventually.

Reference

[1] Otto Kroeger with Janet M. Thuesen, *Type Talk at Work* (New York: Delacorte Press, 1992), p. 395.

Bibliography

Barnhouse, Ruth Tiffany. *Identity* (Philadelphia: Westminister Press, 1984).

Barr, Browne. *High-Flying Geese* (New York: Seabury Press, 1973).

Bolles, Richard Nelson. *What Color Is Your Parachute?* (Berkley, Calif.: Ten Speed Press, 1998).

Bolman, Lee G., and Terrence E. Deal. *Leading with Soul* (San Francisco: Jossey-Bass, 1995).

Brussat, Fredric, and Mary Ann Brussat. *100 Ways to Keep Your Soul Alive, Living Deeply and Fully Every Day* (San Francisco: HarperSanFrancisco, 1994).

Campbell, Joseph. *The Hero with a Thousand Faces* (Princeton, N.J.: Princeton University Press, 1949).

Campbell, Joseph, with Bill Moyers. *The Power of Myth* (New York: Doubleday, 1988).

Chappell, Tom. *The Soul of a Business* (New York: Bantam Books, 1993).

Claremont de Castillejo, Irene. *Knowing Woman* (New York: Harper & Row, 1973).

Corbin, Carolyn. *Conquering Corporate Codependence* (Engelwood Cliffs, N.J.: Prentice Hall Trade, 1993).

DeFoore, Bill, and John Renesch, eds. *Rediscovering the Soul of Business* (San Francisco: New Leaders Press, 1995).

Dossey, Larry, M.D. *Healing Words* (San Francisco: HarperSan-Francisco, 1993).

———. *Meaning and Medicine* (New York: Bantam Books, 1991).

———. *Recovering the Soul* (New York: Bantam Books, 1989).

———. *Space, Time and Medicine* (Boulder, Colo.: New Science Library, 1982).

Finney, Martha, and Deborah Dasch. *Find Your Calling, Love Your Life* (New York: Simon & Schuster, 1998).

Fox, Matthew. *The Reinvention of Work* (New York: HarperCollins, 1994).

Gordon, James S. *Manifesto for a New Medicine, Your Guide to Healing Partnerships and the Wise Use of Alternative Therapies* (New York: Addison-Wesley, 1996).

Gozdz, Kazimierz, ed. *Community Building in Business* (San Francisco: New Leaders Press, 1995).

Hammond, Sue Annis. *The Thin Book of Appreciative Inquiry* (Plano, Tex.: Kodiak Consulting, 1996).

Hesselbein, Frances, Marshall Goldsmith, and Richard Beckhard, eds. The Peter F. Drucker Foundation. *The Community of the Future* (San Francisco: Jossey-Bass, 1998)

Hutschnecker, Arnold A. *The Will to Live* (New York: Cornerstone Library, 1978).

Hyde, Lewis. *The Gift, Imagination and the Erotic Life of Property* (New York: Vintage Books, 1979).

Jaworski, Joseph. *Synchronicity* (San Francisco: Berrett-Koehler Publishers, 1996).

Johnson, Robert. *HE* (King of Prussia, Pa.: Religious Publishing Co., 1974).

———. *SHE* (King of Prussia, Pa.: Religious Publishing Co., 1976).

Jung, C. G., *Letters.* Edited by G. Adler and A. Jaffe. Translated by R. F. C. Hull (Princeton, N.J.: Princeton University Press, 1973).

Lowery, Joan E. *CultureShift* (Chicago: AHA Press, 1997).

Miller, Robert. *Your Golden Shadow* (San Francisco: Harper & Row, 1989).

Moore, Thomas. *Care of the Soul* (New York: HarperCollins, 1992).

———. *Soulmates* (New York: HarperCollins, 1994).

———. *The Reenchantment of Ordinary Life* (New York: Harper-Collins, 1996).

Needleman, Jacob. *Time and the Soul* (New York: Currency/Doubleday, 1998).

Parker, Roy. *Medicine, a History of Healing* (New York: Barnes & Noble, 1997).

Peck, M. Scott. *The Different Drum* (New York: Touchstone, 1987).

———. *The Road Less Traveled* (New York: Simon & Schuster, 1978).

Pulley, Mary Lynn. *Losing Your Job—Reclaiming Your Soul* (San Francisco: Jossey-Bass, 1997).

Ray, Michael, and Rochele Myers. *Creativity in Business* (New York: Doubleday, 1989).

Remen, Rachel Naomi. *Kitchen Table Wisdom* (New York: Riverhead Books, 1996).

Rubin, Irwin M., and Raymond Fernandez. *My Pulse Is Not What It Used To Be, The Leadership Challenges In Health Care* (Honolulu: The Temenos Foundation, 1991).

Ryan, Kathleen D., and Daniel K. Oestreich. *Driving Fear Out of the Workplace* (San Francisco: Jossey-Bass, 1991).

Sanford, John. *Healing and Wholeness* (New York: Paulist Press, 1977).

————. *Soul Journey* (New York: Crossroad, 1991).

Selye, Hans. *Stress without Distress* (New York: New American Library, 1974).

Singer, June. *Boundaries of the Soul* (Garden City, N.Y.: Anchor Books, 1973).

Stone, Richard. *Nightime Stories* (Salt Lake City: Nightime Pediatrics Press, 1998).

Index